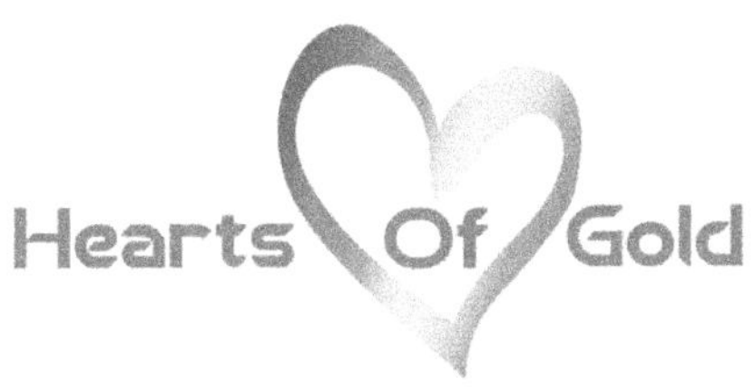

HEARTS OF GOLD

Reflections of

HEALTH

Gold Award Girl Scouts

Sheryl M Robinson

Copyright Page

Published by Grow and Share Network, LLC
First Edition, 2026

ISBN: 978-1-972135-02-0

Printed in the United States of America

Books in the Hearts of Gold Series

- *Earth Guardian*
- *STEM*
- *Creative Voice*
- *Health*
- *Inclusion*
- *Advocacy*
- *Community Connector*

Table of Contents

Chapter 1
Ignite Your Impact!

Every Great Mission Begins with a Single Spark

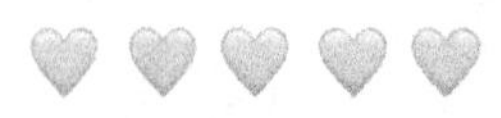

If you slow down and really pay attention to your life, you might notice things that seem small at first. A friend who always feels stressed before school. A classmate who misses days because they're sick. A family member who seems tired, worried, or overwhelmed often. These moments are easy to brush off. Everyone has bad days, right?

But to a Wellness Champion, these moments aren't small at all.

They're signals.

There are clues that something in the world isn't working the way it should — and that someone might need support.

Health isn't just about hospitals, doctors, or emergencies. It's about how people feel day to day. It's about whether students feel safe asking for help, whether families understand what's happening to their bodies or minds, and whether communities have the tools they need to stay well.

Across the country, girls just like you are noticing these clues. They are listening closely to what's happening around them and asking thoughtful questions: Why does this keep happening? Who is being affected? What could make this better?

In this book, you'll meet girls who followed their concern for physical, mental, and emotional health and turned it into action. Their stories prove something powerful:

You don't have to be a doctor to make a difference. You can start right now.

Caring for Minds and Bodies

Some Wellness Champions focus on helping people feel stronger, calmer, and safer in their own bodies and minds.

You'll read about girls who noticed how much stress and anxiety were affecting students their age. They saw classmates struggling silently, unsure how to explain what they were feeling or where to turn for help. Instead of assuming someone else would fix it, these girls stepped up.

They taught peers simple ways to manage stress. They created clear, honest resources that explained mental health without judgment or shame. They opened conversations that helped others realize they weren't alone.

Other Wellness Champions focused on physical health. They noticed classmates who didn't understand how their bodies worked or why certain habits mattered. They saw confusion around nutrition, sleep, exercise, and illness — and responded with education, encouragement, and creativity.

Each of these girls noticed someone struggling and asked an important question: "What could help?"

Then they took action.

Supporting Health

Other Wellness Champions looked beyond their immediate circles and noticed challenges affecting entire communities.

Some saw families overwhelmed by serious or long-term illnesses. Others noticed how little information was available — or how hard it was to talk openly about certain conditions. Some recognized that caregivers often felt isolated, exhausted, and unseen.

Instead of turning away, these girls leaned in.

They created programs to support patients and caregivers. They shared information that people didn't know how to ask for. They helped break the stigma around physical and mental health by talking honestly and respectfully.

These projects weren't always easy. Health topics can be personal. Conversations can feel uncomfortable. Plans don't always work the first time.

But these girls kept going.

They learned how to research carefully, talk to experts, and listen to people with lived experience. They adjusted their plans when obstacles appeared. They discovered that helping others requires patience, empathy, and persistence.

Through their efforts, communities felt more informed, more supported, and more hopeful.

What Makes a Wellness Champion?

Wellness Champions share a few important strengths.

First, they pay attention.

They notice when something doesn't feel right and refuse to ignore it just because it's common or inconvenient. They understand that noticing a problem is the first step toward solving it.

Second, they learn before they act.

They ask questions. They research. They talk to doctors, counselors, teachers, and community leaders. They listen carefully to the people most affected.

Wellness Champions know that good intentions aren't enough — understanding matters.

Third, they believe caring leads to change.

They believe that small actions can grow into a big impact. That one conversation can lead to another. That one project can help many people.

Being a Wellness Champion isn't about perfection.
It's about noticing a need and caring enough to
respond.

You Belong in This Story Too

As you read the chapters ahead, you'll meet girls
who never thought of themselves as health leaders
or advocates.

- They were students. Athletes. Artists. Friends.
- They were busy. Sometimes unsure. Sometimes
  nervous about speaking up.
- What they shared wasn't confidence — it was a
  choice.

They chose not to ignore the signals they noticed.
They chose to learn rather than look away.
They chose to try, even when the outcome wasn't
guaranteed.

- Maybe your passion is mental health.
- Maybe it's illness prevention, nutrition, or healthy
  habits.
- Maybe it's helping people feel supported,
  understood, and less alone.

Whatever makes your heart beat faster — that's
where your journey begins.

This book is full of ideas, courage, and real examples from girls who cared deeply and acted boldly.

🤍 People need care. And you are ready.

Chapter 2
Stretch Out Stress

Marissa Fletcher (Ep 20)

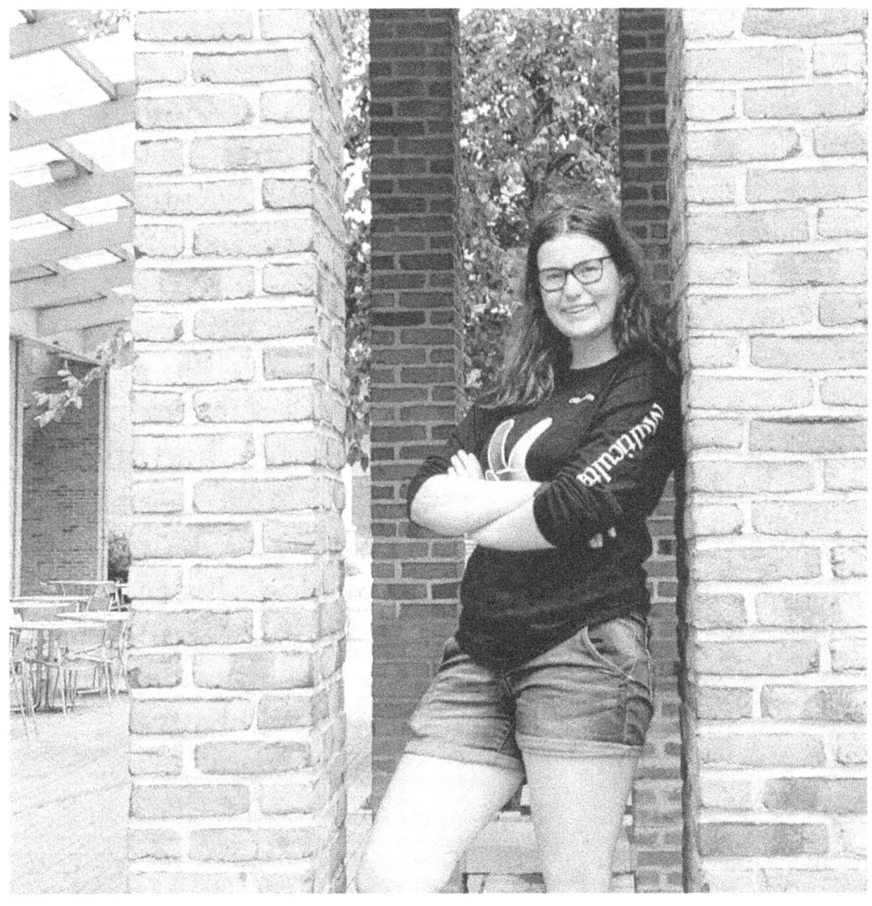

The Weight of the World

For many young people, life is a balancing act of school, friends, and hobbies. But for Marissa Fletcher, the world became very heavy at a very young age. When she was only twelve years old, her mother—who was not only her parent but also her beloved troop leader—passed away unexpectedly. The loss was a devastating blow that rippled through every part of her life. While other middle schoolers were worried about homework or sports, Marissa was navigating a sea of grief and the sudden absence of the woman who had guided her since she was a little girl.

The human body has a strange way of reacting to deep emotional pain. Between her first and second years of high school, the stress of the loss began to manifest in a frightening physical way: Marissa started having non-epileptic seizures. These episodes looked like regular seizures, but they were caused by the intense mental and emotional pressure she was carrying. At the height of her struggle, she was having these seizures up to seven times a day. She was missing classes and losing her sense of control over her own body. The doctors were clear: the seizures were the result of accumulated stress. She needed a way to help her brain and body relax before the damage became permanent.

It was her high school counselor who suggested a solution that seemed, at first, a bit unusual to a teenager. She recommended that Marissa try yoga. Initially, Marissa was skeptical. She had always associated yoga with "older people" and didn't think it could help someone her age. However, she was desperate to stop the seizures and reclaim her life. When she finally stepped onto a mat and began breathing and moving, everything changed. She discovered that yoga allowed her brain to relax while her body got the exercise it needed—a combination that proved to be a powerful weapon against the stress that had been making her sick. This personal healing journey eventually became the spark for her most important project: "Yoga Out of Stress".

Designing the Sanctuary

Once Marissa experienced the life-changing benefits of yoga and meditation, she knew she couldn't keep the secret to herself. She wanted to turn her personal victory into a community mission to help other students who might be silently drowning in their own stress. She decided to launch an initiative to teach yoga and meditation to elementary and high school students in her hometown. But moving from being a yoga student to a teacher was a massive undertaking that required careful planning and a lot of support from her community.

Marissa's first step was to find a mentor who could help her navigate the complicated world of school administration and project management. She turned back to the person who had first suggested yoga to her—her high school counselor. The counselor stepped into a dual role, acting as both her professional advisor and her personal cheerleader. Together, they began to map out how a high school student could realistically teach classes at multiple schools while still maintaining a full academic load. Marissa had to prove that she was dedicated, even when the logistics became overwhelming.

The planning phase was filled with obstacles that tested Marissa's patience. Coordinating the schedules of multiple schools was a giant puzzle. She didn't just have to find time in her own day; she had to align her advisor's schedule with the availability of school facilities. She often found that the gym—the perfect place for a large yoga session—was constantly booked for varsity sports or other school events. There were many days when she felt like she was playing an endless game of phone tag with school principals and athletic directors.

During the most frustrating moments, when it felt like her project might never get off the ground, Marissa would look back at the very first notes she had written during her brainstorming sessions. She reminded herself of why she started: to ensure that no other child had to experience the physical toll of stress alone. By focusing on her "why," she found the strength to keep pushing through the "how." She learned that leadership isn't just about having a great idea; it's about the grit required to manage a calendar and keep your ducks in a row when everything feels like it's falling apart.

The Mats Are Out

The execution of the "Yoga Out of Stress" project was a beautiful display of community and movement. Marissa moved from school to school, carrying a message of peace and health to students of all ages. She quickly realized that you can't teach a seven-year-old the same way you teach a seventeen-year-old. To make her initiative successful, she had to tailor her curriculum to fit the energy of each group she visited. The elementary schoolers were a highlight for her; they brought a wild, infectious enthusiasm to every session, making the "work" feel like a celebration.

To ensure her sessions were both fun and effective, Marissa utilized several key resources and partnerships throughout the community:

High School Counselor Advisor: This mentor provided the professional guidance needed to format the stress-relief curriculum and provided moral support when the workload grew heavy.

Local School Facilities: Marissa partnered with both her local elementary school and high school to provide free space for the classes, navigating complex gym-sharing schedules.

Peer-to-Peer Feedback: She constantly collected feedback from her students to ensure her meditation tips and yoga poses were easy to understand and truly helpful for their age groups.

As she led the classes, Marissa explained to the students how yoga works to calm the mind. She taught them that by focusing on their breath and the way their muscles moved, they were permitting their brains to "relax". She shared specific meditation tips they could use right at their desks before a big test or after a tough day. Seeing the students close their eyes and find a moment of quiet in their busy school days was the ultimate reward for the months of planning.

However, even as she taught others to stay calm, Marissa had to practice what she preached. She was still a busy student herself, and she had to learn how to manage her time so that her project didn't become a source of the very stress she was trying to fight. This project taught her that being a leader means being a role model. She couldn't tell students to prioritize their mental health if she wasn't doing the same. By the time her final class ended, Marissa hadn't just taught yoga—she had built a movement of mindfulness that had truly taken root in her small town.

Unexpected "Thank You"

The true impact of a project often isn't seen the moment the final report is signed. For Marissa, the proof of her success came in small, quiet moments long after her classes had ended. Her community didn't just participate in the classes and move on; they carried her lessons into their daily lives. The most visible sign of this was a professional job offer: because of the success of her project, Marissa was offered a position teaching yoga at the local Boys and Girls Club. Her "volunteer" project had turned into a career opportunity before she had even finished school.

One afternoon, about a year after she had finished her project, Marissa was sitting on the bus on her way home. A little girl approached her with wide eyes and a look of recognition. "You're that girl," the child said. When Marissa asked what she meant, the girl replied, "You're the girl that did yoga at my school. Because of you, I started doing yoga on a daily basis". In that moment, sitting on a noisy bus, Marissa realized that her mission was truly completed. She had changed the life of at least one person, giving them a tool for health that they would use for years to come.

The impact also reached far beyond the yoga mats. Marissa's dedication to her project led to incredible opportunities for her future. She was featured on a national blog, sharing her story about how her years of service helped her earn enough scholarships to pay for her first year and a half of college without taking on any loans. The post went viral, receiving over 140 comments and thousands of likes. People from all over were inspired by the girl from a small town who had turned a personal tragedy into a national success story.

Reflecting on her journey, Marissa realized that the skills she gained weren't just about yoga. She had learned how to manage a team, speak in public, and communicate with people with very different points of view. But most importantly, she learned the power of the "ripple effect." One girl deciding to share her healing journey had led to hundreds of students learning meditation, a little girl on a bus finding a daily healthy habit, and a national audience seeing the potential of young leaders to change the world.

Building a Lifetime of Strength

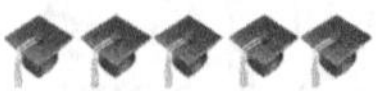

As Marissa moved into her college years, she looked back on her time with great pride. She realized that her project was only the final chapter of a journey that began when she was a young child. She had learned the building blocks of success years earlier, in middle school, where she was taught how to budget, save money, and keep logs of her finances to prepare for trips. These practical skills enabled her to manage her scholarships so well that she could attend college without the burden of debt.

Her years in Girl Scouts were filled with more than just work; they were filled with memories that made the hard times easier to bear. She fondly remembered horseback riding on the slowest horse in the group, with her mom at the very front and twenty other girls in between. She cherished the memories of creek-hopping, camping for a week at a time, and the "mom and me" classes, where she spent precious hours with her mother. She even got to travel to California and Disney World as a chaperone for younger girls, proving that she had transitioned from a student to a trusted leader.

Marissa's biggest piece of advice for any girl starting her own journey is simple but profound: never give up. There were many moments when she felt discouraged, especially during the planning phase when it seemed like no one's schedule would align. She knew that her mom had earned her Gold Award, and that legacy kept her moving forward even when she wanted to quit. She learned that if you find your passion and work with it, the hours will go by in a flash, and the reward at the end will be worth every sacrifice. Marissa Fletcher moves forward with the quiet, steady strength of someone who knows exactly how to find the calm in any storm.

Chapter 3
Clearing the Air

Aria Chalileh (Ep 61)

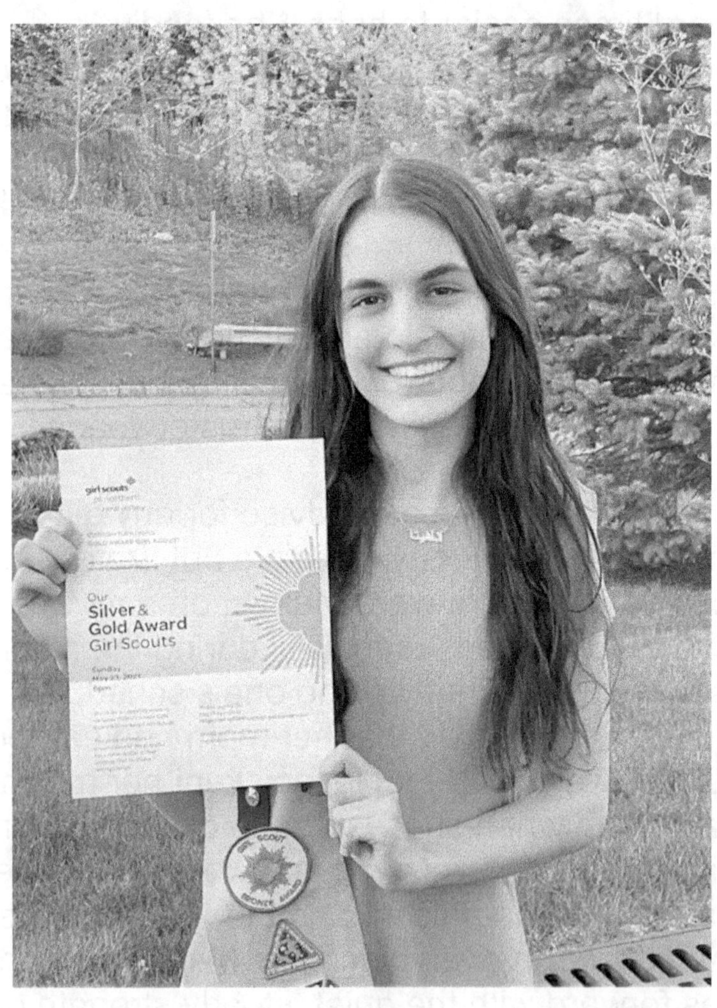

Foundation of Service

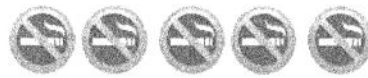

For Aria Chalileh, the journey toward leadership didn't begin with a single grand gesture, but rather with a series of small, dedicated steps that started when she was only in the second grade. Growing up in Bergen County, New Jersey, she spent years in Girl Scouts, learning the value of community and the importance of lending a hand to those in need. One of her earliest memories of taking action was in the fifth grade, during her elementary school years, when she worked with her troop to host a "pet day in the park". This early project was designed to be environmentally friendly and encouraged local families to get outside and enjoy the natural world together. It was through these early experiences that Aria began to understand that even a young girl could organize an event that brought people together for a good cause.

As she moved into middle school, Aria's sense of responsibility toward her community continued to grow, leading her to tackle her Girl Scout Silver Award with an oral cancer awareness project. This was a topic close to home, as her mother worked in a related medical field and had always been passionate about the issue. Aria realized through her research that while many types of cancer receive public attention, oral cancer is often overlooked by the general public. She spent her time creating brochures and pamphlets, attending local events, and educating her community about the risks associated with smoking. This experience was a crucial building block, teaching her how to research complex medical topics and translate them into information that regular people could understand.

When Aria finally reached high school, she noticed a troubling shift in the environment around her. Years earlier, she and her peers had gone through the DARE program, which taught them about the dangers of drugs and alcohol at a young age. However, as they grew older, many of those same peers began using new and dangerous products that hadn't been a major part of the conversation when they were children: vaping devices. Aria saw that the vaping epidemic was not just a national crisis, but a local one affecting her friends and classmates in New Jersey. She felt a deep, personal pull to address this youth vaping epidemic, realizing that her previous work with oral cancer had provided her with the perfect transition into this new, more urgent mission. She decided that her project would be dedicated to clearing the air and protecting the health of her generation.

The Vaping Crisis

Transitioning from oral cancer awareness to vaping prevention felt like a natural evolution for Aria, as both issues were rooted in the dangers of traditional and electronic smoking. She understood that to make a real difference, she couldn't just tell her peers that vaping was "bad"; she had to understand the "why" behind the epidemic. She began a deep dive into the root causes of why students were turning to these devices in the first place. Her research revealed a complex web of factors, including the aggressive marketing practices of big tobacco companies and the intense peer pressure that many teenagers feel to fit in with their social groups. She also discovered that many students used vaping to cope with stress, seeking the "buzz" or the feeling of relief that the nicotine provided.

Aria realized that tobacco companies were specifically targeting youth through their marketing, and she wanted to shift the narrative away from blaming students. Instead of wagging a finger at her classmates, she wanted to empower them with the most up-to-date information so they could make well-informed decisions. She joined several advocacy groups focused on vaping prevention and awareness to deepen her knowledge and connect with others fighting the same battle. This collaborative spirit helped her realize that she wasn't alone in her concerns and that a united voice would be much more powerful than a solo effort.

Being a debater and someone who genuinely enjoyed public speaking, Aria knew that her voice was her strongest tool. She had spent years standing up for what she believed in, but addressing a "taboo" topic like vaping brought a new set of nerves. She knew that many of the people she would be presenting to were likely using the very products she was speaking against. However, Aria's passion for the cause outweighed her fear of rejection. She believed that if she could reach even one person and help them choose a healthier path, the entire effort would be worth it. She set out to create a curriculum that didn't just list health hazards but offered alternatives— teaching her peers to "choose a natural buzz" and find healthier ways to manage the stresses of high school life. This mindset of empowerment through education became the heartbeat of her mission.

Blueprint for Change

Once Aria had a firm grasp of the research and a clear vision for her message, she began the hard work of building the infrastructure for her project. She knew that to maximize her outreach, she needed to meet people where they were—in the classrooms, on their phones, and in the local news. She didn't want this to be a one-time speech; she wanted to create a lasting set of resources that the county could use long after she graduated. She began reaching out to middle and high schools throughout Bergen County, coordinating with administrators to schedule speaking engagements with students. This required immense organization and a detailed action plan to ensure every presentation was professional and impactful.

The core of her strategy was the "peer-to-peer" approach. Aria realized that teenagers are much more likely to listen to someone their own age who understands their world than to an adult who might seem disconnected from current trends. She used her knowledge of what was "trendy" and what youth liked to make her presentations engaging and relatable. She wasn't just a girl giving a lecture; she was a classmate sharing vital information that could save lives. To ensure her message reached as many people as possible, Aria followed a specific plan of action:

County-Wide Presentations: She conducted multiple educational sessions at various middle and high schools across Bergen County to address health consequences and peer pressure.

Digital Media Creation: She produced a short, high-impact YouTube video to share prevention facts in a format easy for youth to watch and share.

Public Advocacy Journalism: She wrote a detailed article about the vaping epidemic to provide a written resource for those who preferred reading over watching videos.

Resource Integration: She partnered with school student assistance counselors to provide "quit resources" for students who were already struggling with nicotine addiction.

Aria's ability to coordinate these different moving parts was a testament to her leadership growth. She was also very active as the community outreach leader for her high school robotics team, where she helped brainstorm events to encourage younger kids to get involved in STEAM. This experience organizing large-scale events, such as a STEAM fair with 30 booths, gave her the confidence to manage the logistics of her vaping prevention project. She learned that whether you are talking about 3D printers or the dangers of nicotine, the key to a successful project is staying organized and having a team that believes in the mission. Aria spent countless hours refining her slides and practicing her delivery, ensuring that she was prepared for any question that might come her way.

Navigating a Virtual World

Just as Aria's project was gaining significant momentum, an unexpected and global challenge appeared: the pandemic. Like many other girls working on their projects, Aria found that the world she knew had suddenly shut down. The in-person presentations she had worked so hard to organize were no longer possible, and the schools were closed to outside visitors. At first, this felt like a major setback that could have stalled her mission entirely. However, Aria realized that the stress of the pandemic might make the vaping crisis worse, as more youth might turn to these products to cope with the isolation and anxiety of quarantine.

Instead of giving up, Aria showed the resilience of a true leader by pivoting her entire strategy to a virtual setting. She began utilizing tools like Zoom and Google Meet to conduct her presentations remotely. While she missed the energy of being in a room with her peers, she soon discovered an unexpected benefit of the digital shift. Being virtual allowed her to reach people across the country who might not have been able to attend an in-person event. Her outreach expanded, proving that sometimes a detour can lead to an even better destination. She adapted her presentations to include interactive games and strategies that worked in a digital format, ensuring that the "peer-to-peer" connection remained strong even through a screen.

Another major challenge was the nature of the topic itself. Vaping was a "taboo" subject, and Aria often faced resistance from people who did not like being told to quit. She had to find a way to be vocal and stand her ground without alienating the very people she was trying to help. She learned to navigate these difficult social waters by focusing on the "big tobacco" companies as the villains, rather than the students who were using the products. By providing resources and directing her peers to student assistance counselors, she offered a hand of support rather than a finger of blame. This empathetic approach enabled her to connect with diverse audiences, even those initially skeptical of her message. Through the "virtual fog" of the pandemic, Aria's voice remained a clear and steady guide for her community.

Advocate to Leader

The impact of Aria's project was both visible and measurable, with feedback surveys showing that 85% to 95% of her audience found the information helpful and intended to apply the lessons to their own lives. She successfully raised awareness of tobacco companies' marketing tactics and empowered her peers to seek a "natural buzz" rather than a chemical one. For Aria, completing this project felt like the end of a major chapter in her life, one that had transformed her from a shy second-grader into a confident advocate for her generation. She had learned that she didn't need to be an adult to make a difference; she just needed to be organized and passionate about her cause.

Her leadership growth throughout the project was immense. She overcame her fear of rejection and learned to be vocal about a difficult subject, benefiting her entire community. These skills were not just for her current project but for her entire life. Aria set her sights on the next stage of her journey: attending the College of New Jersey. Her experiences in debate and public advocacy led her to choose a political science major on a pre-law track. She hopes to attend law school eventually and either become an attorney or run for public office, where she can continue to use her voice to shape legislation and help others on a larger scale.

Aria's advice to younger girls who are considering their own project is simple: "Get organized. " She emphasizes the importance of having an action plan and choosing a topic you are truly passionate about before you even start the proposal process. She knows firsthand that things won't always go exactly as imagined, but being able to "pivot" is one of the most valuable lessons a leader can learn. Aria's journey proved that with a clear vision and the courage to speak up, one girl can challenge an entire industry and clear the air for those around her.

Aria Chalileh's mission was to break through the thick clouds of the vaping epidemic, and she did so by providing her peers with the sunlight of truth. Her project was like a steady wind that pushed away the "taboo" fog, revealing a path toward health and self-informed choices. As she moves forward into her career in law and politics, Aria carries with her the knowledge that she has already made a lasting impact, one presentation and one clear breath at a time.

Chapter 4
Out of the Darkness

Kyra Berry (Ep 98)

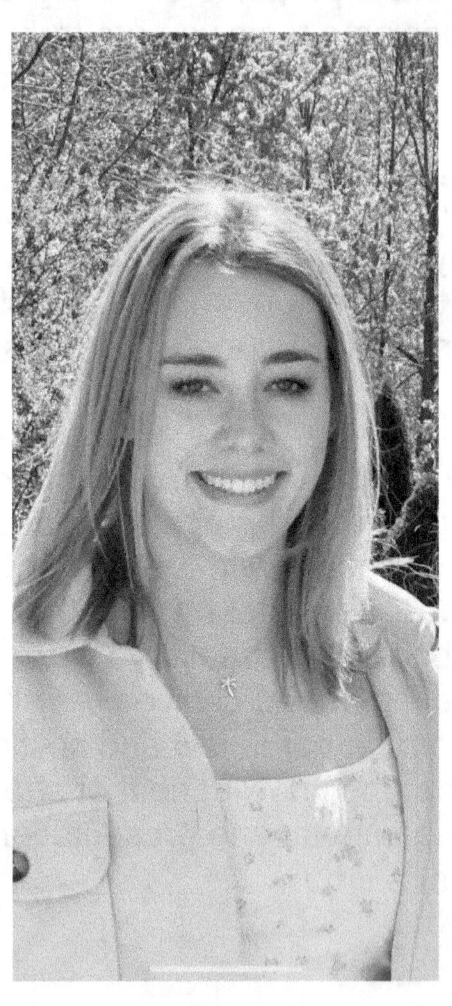

Silence of the Heart

Kyra Berry's journey into leadership began during a time that felt anything but bright. When she was just thirteen years old, she was diagnosed with depression, a struggle that stayed with her through every year of high school. There was a time when the weight of her mental health was so heavy that she couldn't even make it through a full day of classes. Her mother often had to pick her up from school early because she was hurting so much. During those difficult days, Kyra realized that a major part of the pain was the silence surrounding mental illness. She felt as though she had to hide the truth and tell people she was struggling with something else entirely. This feeling of having to lie or stay quiet created a barrier between her and her community that she desperately wanted to break.

As she began to feel better, a new sense of purpose took root. She looked back at the incredible support she had received from her family and her school during her darkest moments and felt a deep surge of gratitude. She knew that no one should ever have to feel alone or ashamed of what they were going through. Kyra decided that her leadership project should tackle the very thing she had faced: the stigma of mental health. She wanted to create a space where people could talk openly and find the tools they needed to manage the pressure of daily life.

Kyra's motivation was simple: she wanted to give back to the community that had carried her through her own storm. She knew that by sharing her own story, she could help others realize that it is truly okay not to be okay. Her project wasn't just about finishing a requirement; it was a personal mission to transform her struggle into a beacon of hope for her peers. She was ready to step out of her comfort zone and lead, not just for herself, but for every other student who was still sitting in the heavy silence.

Planting Seeds of Calm

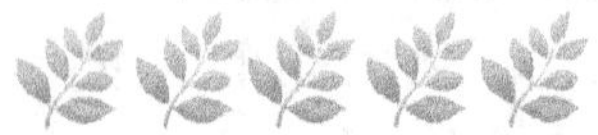

To address the stress she saw in her high school hallways, Kyra decided to launch the "Stress Less Club". She knew that high school was a pressure cooker of exams, social drama, and future worries, and she wanted to give her classmates practical ways to find their center. She envisioned a club that wasn't just another boring meeting, but a localized effort to educate her peers about how stress affects the brain and how to fight back against it. Kyra wanted to bring in experts to show that wellness could be found in many different places, from the food we eat to the way we move our bodies.

Getting the club started was a massive task that required Kyra to think like a professional organizer. She had to prove there was a genuine need for such a group and that it wouldn't just overlap with other activities already offered at the school. She drafted a formal plan and worked closely with her English teacher, who shared her wellness mindset and agreed to be her advisor. Together, they navigated the long approval process required by the school administration. To get the mission moving, Kyra focused on several key steps to ensure her project was carried out correctly:

Identifying a teacher advisor who understands the daily stressors high schoolers face.
Gathering a list of at least fifteen interested students to show the school board that people wanted this club.
Developing a curriculum for weekly meetings that included guest speakers and hands-on activities.
Creating digital signage and eye-catching posters to advertise the club's inaugural meeting throughout the school building.

The hard work paid off in a way Kyra never expected. When the doors opened for the very first meeting, nearly forty students walked in. It was a powerful moment that proved Kyra wasn't the only one feeling the weight of the world; her peers were also looking for a way to manage their stress. Every week, she brought in different professionals to share their time. A dietician from a local grocery store came to talk about foods that boost your mood, while other experts taught yoga, meditation, or even art classes designed to promote calm. Kyra had successfully turned her school from a place of high-stakes pressure into a sanctuary where her friends could finally breathe.

Path Through Darkness

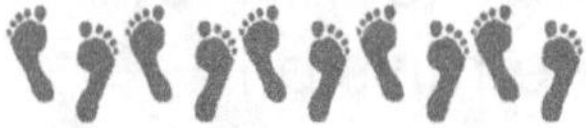

While the club was making a difference at school, Kyra felt a pull to do something even bigger for her entire county. She decided that the second part of her project would be to organize a suicide prevention walk. She had seen how powerful it was for people to come together for a common cause, and she wanted to create a day dedicated to hope and healing. Kyra didn't have any experience in event planning, so she did what many great leaders do: she started with a search engine. She looked for organizations specializing in mental health walks and found the American Foundation for Suicide Prevention (AFSP).

Partnering with the AFSP turned out to be an incredible experience for Kyra. She learned that anyone could start a walk in their community if they were willing to put in the work. Though she was only sixteen years old at the time, she dove into the complicated paperwork required to make the walk an official event. She had to figure out everything from the route of the walk to the legal permissions needed to host a large public gathering. Kyra's family stepped up to support her, helping her find her footing and build a team that could turn her vision into a reality.

The very first "Out of the Darkness Walk" in Burlington County was small, but it was deeply meaningful. Kyra stood at the starting line and realized that she had created a space where people could honor their loved ones and share their own stories without fear of judgment. The event gave the community a chance to publicly break the stigma that Kyra had once struggled with in private. It was more than just a walk; it was a physical representation of people moving together from a place of pain toward a place of light. By leading this massive effort, Kyra proved that a single girl with a clear goal can mobilize an entire community to support one another.

Paperwork Mountain

Building a lasting movement was not without its roadblocks, and Kyra often felt like she was climbing a mountain made of red tape. The paperwork process to get her high school club approved was surprisingly long and tedious. She had to carefully explain why her club deserved a spot in the school's busy schedule and convince the administration that her ideas were sound. There were times when she had to draft and re-draft her proposals, proving that her persistence was just as important as her passion. This taught her that being a leader often means spending as much time with pen and paper as with people.

Another major challenge was the walk itself, which required planning that began as early as January for an event in October. Balancing the heavy workload of her junior and senior years of high school with the constant needs of the walk was a true test of her resilience. She had to learn how to communicate her vision to local business owners to ask for sponsorships, which felt intimidating at first.

When the walk happened in 2021, the community came in droves. The isolation of the pandemic had made mental health a top priority for everyone, and people were more eager than ever to connect. Kyra realized that the "speed bumps" she encountered—the paperwork, the long hours—were all part of the learning process. She learned to handle problems that once seemed insurmountable and discovered that her voice could reach politicians and business leaders alike. Her project taught her that true leadership isn't about avoiding obstacles, but about having the grit to keep walking until the path clears.

Seven Year Legacy

The impact of Kyra's project didn't stop when she graduated from high school; it grew as she became a young adult. The walk she started as a junior is still going strong seven years later. In 2022, the 7th annual Burlington County Out of the Darkness Walk raised over $52,000, a number Kyra found almost unbelievable to say out loud. Local politicians now come to speak at the event, and her hometown of Mount Laurel even issued a proclamation honoring September as suicide prevention month because of her efforts. Kyra has watched people travel from other states just to be part of the community she built.

Completing her project changed the way Kyra viewed herself and her future. She graduated from Loyola University Maryland with a degree in communications and double minors in political science and marketing. She works in crisis communications at an advertising agency in Philadelphia, using the skills she gained during her project to manage the reputations and issues of various organizations. She realized that the networking, public speaking, and resilience she practiced while earning her award were the perfect foundation for a professional career. Even with a busy job, Kyra remains part of the leadership team for the annual walk, considering it her favorite volunteer work.

Looking back, Kyra credits much of her growth to the sisterhood she found in Girl Scouts. Having her mother as her troop leader for thirteen years helped them form a deep bond that she still values today. She encourages any girl considering a big project to follow a cause they truly care about, because that passion will be the fuel they need when the work gets tough. Kyra started her journey as a girl who felt broken by depression, but she finished it as a leader who helped heal her entire community. Her story is proof that your greatest struggle can become your greatest strength if you are brave enough to share it.

Chapter 5
A Unicorn's Tale

Ripley Cusinato (Ep 113)

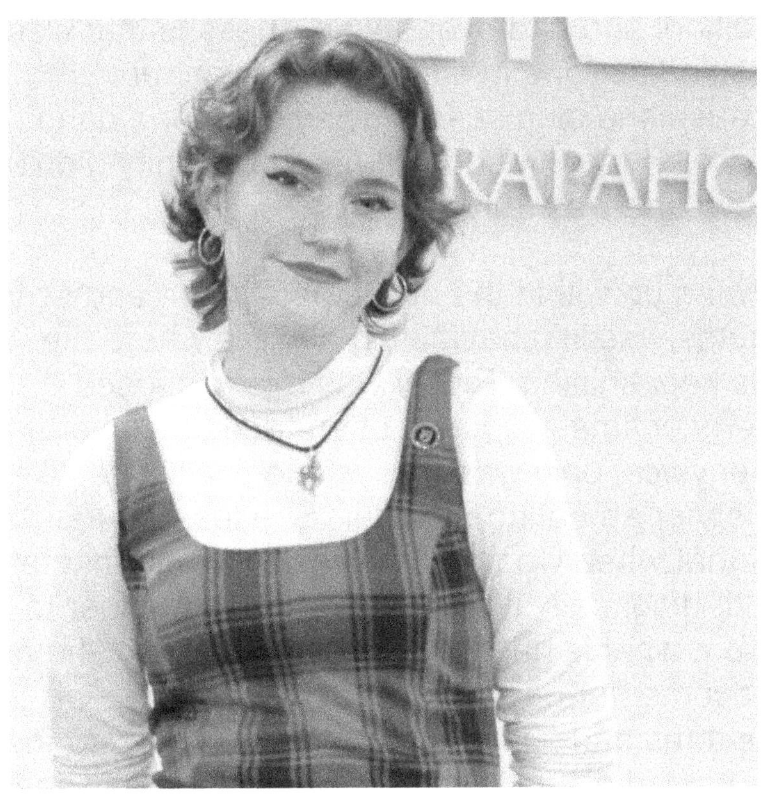

Medical Mystery

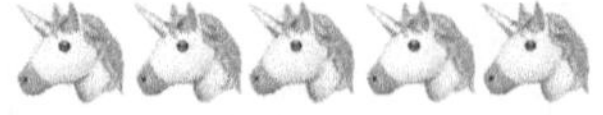

Imagine looking in the mirror and seeing a healthy, normal teenager, yet knowing that, deep inside, your body is fighting a war no one else can see. This was the daily reality for Ripley Cusinato. For years, she lived as a "medical unicorn," a term used for people with conditions so rare they seem like myths. Ripley didn't just have one rare condition; she had over seven illnesses that were classified as "one in a million" or even rarer. Because she didn't use a wheelchair or a cane every day, many people in her community didn't believe she was truly struggling.

Growing up within the public healthcare and school systems was like navigating a maze where the walls kept shifting. Ripley was misdiagnosed dozens of times. Doctors often tried to tell her that her physical pain was a psychological issue, like anxiety or an eating disorder. She learned the hard way that when women receive the wrong mental health diagnosis, it can take five times longer to find out what is happening in their bodies. She had to become her own detective, researching her symptoms and fighting to be heard in a world that only valued disabilities they could physically see.

The turning point came in a creative writing class. Ripley decided to write a final project about a major surgery she had undergone that semester—a surgery that had quite literally saved her life. Her final paper was 27 pages long, triple the required length, because her story was too big to be contained in a few paragraphs. When her professor and classmates read it over a Zoom call, the reaction was immediate and overwhelming. They were appalled by the failures of the medical system but inspired by the fact that Ripley was still standing. "Why haven't you written a book?" they asked her. At first, Ripley doubted herself, wondering who would even care about her journey. But the spark had been lit. She realized her story wasn't just hers; it was a voice for the millions of Americans suffering from chronic illnesses. She decided to turn this mission into her Gold Award.

Ten-Month Race

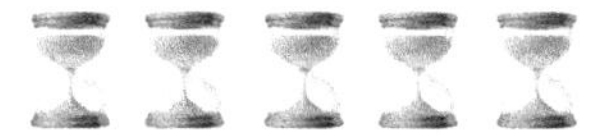

Ripley was not a girl who did things the easy way. Most people spend years writing, editing, and publishing a book, but Ripley didn't have years. She didn't even decide to start her project until she was about to graduate from high school. This left her with a daunting ten-month window before the final deadline. When she approached the council and told them she wanted to write and publish a book in less than a year, they were honest with her. They told her she was a little bit crazy, but they also said that if she believed she could do it, they would support her. That vote of confidence was all she needed to start her engine.

The project requirements demanded that her work be sustainable and impactful. Still, Ripley faced a massive financial hurdle: she wasn't allowed to put any of her own money into the project to fund the publishing. In the literary world, there are two main paths. The traditional route involves finding an agent and a publisher who will pay for editing and marketing. Ripley reached out to over 50 book editors to see if anyone would donate their time. Every single one of them said no, explaining that they usually charge per word, and a full-length book could cost thousands of dollars to polish.

She refused to let a lack of money silence her message. If she couldn't hire a team, she would become the team. She decided to take the self-publishing route, which meant she had to master every single step of the process on her own. This wasn't just about writing anymore; it was about project management and grit. She had to structure her creative process to be incredibly disciplined to hit her deadlines. She spent roughly eight months writing the entire manuscript, but that was only the beginning of the heavy lifting. Every hour spent staring at the computer screen was a step toward proving that her "impossible project" was possible.

Author's Toolbox

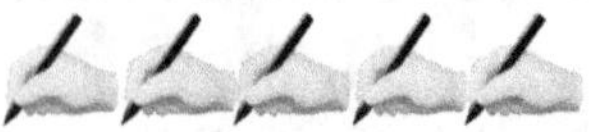

To carry out her project without a single dollar of funding, Ripley transformed into a one-woman publishing house. She didn't have a graphic designer to make her book look professional, so she took graphic design courses to learn the skills herself. She spent 20 hours just designing the cover of her book, making sure it captured the essence of being a "unicorn" in a world that didn't understand her. She also spent over 50 hours on the grueling task of self-editing. Most authors take months off between writing and editing to see their work with fresh eyes, but Ripley had to jump in immediately to stay on schedule.

Because her project needed global reach and to remain active long after she finished, she had to find a tool that was both free and powerful. She chose to work with the Kindle Direct Publishing platform through Amazon. This was a brilliant tactical move because it solved two problems at once: it allowed her to format the book for digital and print use, and it used Amazon's international shipping network to make the book available to readers in other countries without Ripley having to pay for stamps or boxes.

Throughout the process, Ripley used a variety of techniques to maintain high productivity and a sharp focus. To manage the massive amount of work required for her project, she followed a specific set of habits:

Setting a daily word count goal: She committed to writing 1,000 words every single day, regardless of whether she felt inspired or tired.

Using the Pomodoro Method: She worked in focused time blocks, followed by short rewards, such as breaks or snacks, to prevent burnout during long editing sessions.

Applying the "Do Nothing" Rule: On days when she lacked motivation, she gave herself the choice to either write or do absolutely nothing—no phone, no movies, no distractions—until the work got done.

Writing a book about her own trauma was physically and emotionally exhausting. There were mornings when she didn't want to cry or deal with the headache that followed the emotional stress of reliving her medical failures. She had to learn the balance between pushing through like a "toddler throwing a fit" and knowing when her body truly needed a rest. By the time she hit the final "submit" button on Amazon, she had created a polished, 100,000-word piece of art that was entirely her own.

Around The Globe

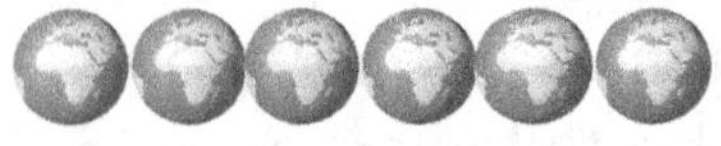

When Ripley's book, *A Unicorn's Childhood*, finally went live, she had modest expectations. She hoped she might sell 50 copies to friends and family. She hadn't spent any money on marketing or hired a publicist to shout her name from the rooftops. But because she had chosen a topic that addressed a massive global need—the understanding of invisible disabilities—the world found her anyway. Three months after her project was finalized, she reviewed the Amazon sales and was absolutely stunned.

She hadn't just reached her local community; she had reached 19 different countries. In an ironic twist of fate, her book was more popular outside of the United States than inside of it. Her most popular country was Germany. Ripley found it fascinating and even a little funny that people on the other side of the Atlantic Ocean were devouring a book about the failures of the American healthcare system. By that three-month mark, she had sold nearly 300 copies purely through people finding it on Google or Amazon. For a young author with no budget, 300 copies was a gigantic, record-breaking number.

The impact of her project wasn't just about the numbers; it was about the education she provided to those who read her words. She taught readers that "don't judge a book by its cover" applies to humans, too. She used her platform to explain that a person in a wheelchair might still be able to walk, or that the sound of a dishwasher might trigger someone with PTSD. By sharing the intimate details of her journey up to age 18, she redefined what disability looks like for an international audience. Her project became a sustainable resource that continued to sell and educate even while she was busy attending college. She had successfully turned her "invisible" struggle into a very visible beacon of hope for others.

Beyond The Page

Completing this massive project changed Ripley from the inside out. It gave her the confidence to realize that she could be her own boss and lead a complex team of supporters, even if that team was mostly her own determined spirit. She learned that leadership isn't just about giving orders; it's about recognizing the people who help you and having the strength to let go of the people who hurt you. In the final chapters of her book, she made the powerful choice to publicly thank the people who had been positive influences, like her surgeon and her mother, who was also her troop leader. But she also did something even more brave: she chose to let go of the harm caused by unsupportive teachers and bullies. She thanked them, too, because without their negativity, she wouldn't have had such a powerful story to write.

Ripley is focusing on her future, which still includes a lot of ink and paper. She continues to write poetry and creative non-fiction for various literary publications, often focusing on the medical side of life. While she is still fighting her illnesses and facing more surgeries, she is no longer in the "active stages of dying" that she experienced as a younger teen. She is a much healthier version of herself and uses that strength to remain active in her creative writing club and local author showcases. She even dreams of having her book professionally edited one day to take it to the next level.

Her advice to any girl thinking about a big project is to find something you are truly passionate about and start as early as you can. She calls her journey the "impossible project," but she proved that with enough heart and a thousand words a day, the impossible is just a starting line. Ripley's project didn't just end with a medal or a certificate; it ended with a new sense of self. She stepped out of the shadows of her rare diseases and into the spotlight as an advocate, a leader, and a published author.

Chapter 6
Journey of Memories

Valencia Julien (Ep 127)

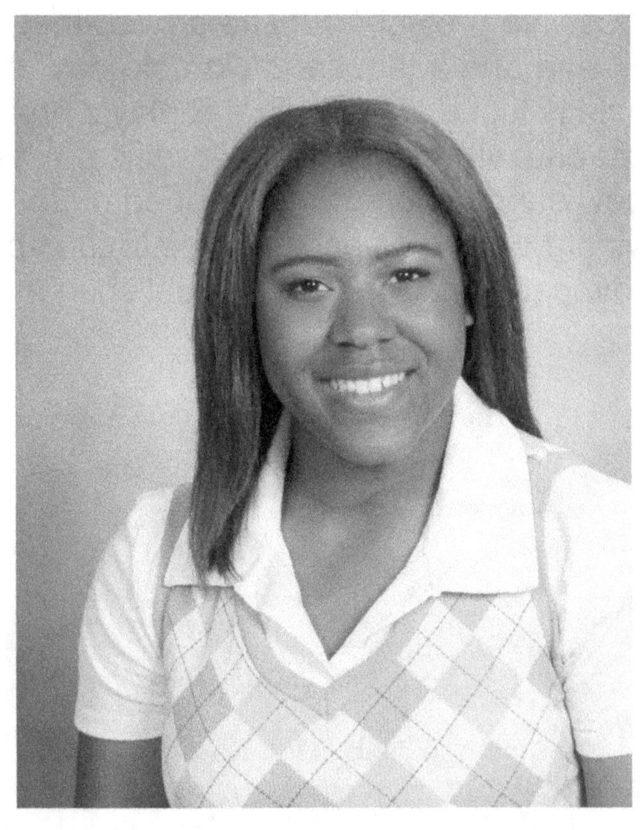

Grandfather's Song

♪♪♪♪♪♪♪♪♪♪♪♪♪

Valencia Julien's journey into leadership did not begin with a checklist or a formal meeting; it started with the sound of piano keys and the steady hum of a car engine. Her grandfather was the primary motivator in her life, a man who had migrated her entire family to a new country with the dream of providing them a better future. As a first-generation student in the US, Valencia carried his pride like a badge of honor. He was the one who drove her to and from school every day, the one who navigated her to her various extracurricular activities, and most importantly, the teacher who sat beside her on the piano bench, guiding her fingers across the keys.

However, when Valencia was in the second grade, a shadow began to fall over their relationship. It started with small lapses in memory, but it quickly evolved into a "huge shift" in their family dynamic. The man who had been her navigator and her musical mentor could no longer drive. Eventually, the most heartbreaking moment of all arrived: he could no longer remember her name. For a young child, this was a terrifying and confusing transformation. Valencia still felt a deep, powerful love for her grandfather, but she realized that maintaining their relationship would now require "work on her end".

As she entered her first year of high school, Valencia knew she wanted to complete her Gold Award, but she struggled to find a topic that felt right. She looked at her theater background and her sports, but nothing clicked until her mother suggested looking interpersonally at the things that had shaped her soul. Alzheimer's disease had made the biggest impact on her life, and she realized that other children were likely feeling the same confusion she had felt back in second grade. She saw a massive gap between the wisdom of older people and the childlike experience of youth. Valencia decided she wanted to be the bridge between those two worlds, transforming her personal grief into a tool that could help thousands of other families navigate the same difficult path.

Writing For A Generation

Valencia envisioned a project that would simplify the complexities of neuroscience for a seven-year-old brain. She decided to create a children's book titled *Giselle Learns about Alzheimer's*. The story follows a young girl named Giselle who discovers her grandmother has the disease and takes it upon herself to learn how to keep their bond strong despite the changes. Valencia didn't just want to write a biography of her own life; she wanted the character to be relatable to as many people as possible. She drew the likeness of the character from a biracial girl she had babysat, knowing that

"Alzheimer's is a disease that doesn't have any racial boundaries".

Building this project was a massive undertaking that required Valencia to go far beyond being just a writer. After her first meeting with an advisor, she received a reality check: she couldn't just publish a book and call it a day. To truly lead, she needed interpersonal connection and community engagement. This meant she had to build a professional team to ensure her medical information was accurate, and her language was appropriate for her young target audience. She reached out to neighborhood community centers and nursing homes, transforming her solitary writing task into a community-wide mission.

To carry out the project effectively, Valencia coordinated with several key partners and followed specific steps to ensure her message reached those in need:

Partnered with the New Jersey Alzheimer's Association to obtain medical pamphlets and goodie bags for session participants.
Collaborated with elementary school teachers to edit the manuscript and ensure the story arc made sense for second and third graders.
Recruited student volunteers to help translate the book into multiple languages, allowing the project to bridge cultural gaps in her community.

Established a YouTube platform to host videos of people reading the book in various languages, ensuring the resources were sustainable and accessible globally.
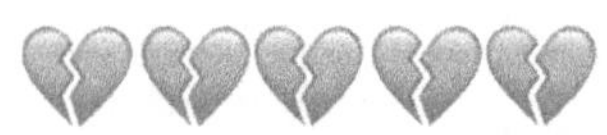

Valencia's mom acted as her personal secretary during this time, helping her manage calls that occurred during the school day or while Valencia was at sports games. Even though she had a team, Valencia remained the clear leader. She learned that while it "takes a village" to create something impactful, she had to be the one to say, "This is what I want, and this is how I want to execute it". She was no longer just a girl who had lost her grandfather to a disease; she was an advocate using her voice to make the world a less confusing place for the next generation of grandchildren.

The Toughest Chapter

💔💔💔

Just as Valencia was preparing to take her book into the community, she faced a challenge that no amount of planning could have prevented. Her grandfather, her biggest motivation and the heart behind the entire project, passed away. His death occurred right after she had published the e-book and received her first batch of printed copies. Suddenly, the project felt devastatingly heavy. She struggled to focus on her schoolwork, and the thought of leading cheerful sessions with children while her heart was breaking felt almost impossible.

The grief was a mountain she had to climb every single day. She had to sit in front of classrooms and read a story that "rang true to my life" and contained fragments of her most painful experiences. There were moments when she wasn't sure she could maintain the "cheer and joy" required to engage second graders. However, Valencia found a way to push through by looking at the bigger picture. She realized that her grandfather would have wanted her to succeed, especially since he had brought the family to the United States specifically so his grandchildren could accomplish great things. She began to see her project as a way to channel her experience into a resource that would prevent other children from feeling the same isolation she had endured.

The pandemic added another layer of difficulty, forcing Valencia to move her in-person sessions to Zoom. She had never met many of her advisors in person, and she found it hard to stay motivated when her entire educational life was happening through a screen. Despite these hurdles, the community's response was overwhelming. When she held her first Zoom session with 40 children at the Morristown Neighborhood House, she saw them leaning in, completely engaged with Giselle's story. Kids began asking her questions, with one even wondering if her own sister had Alzheimer's because she forgot things sometimes. This connection gave Valencia the strength to keep going; she realized that by helping these kids understand the difference between normal forgetting and a serious disease, she was providing them with a sense of safety she hadn't had herself.

Breaking Language Barriers

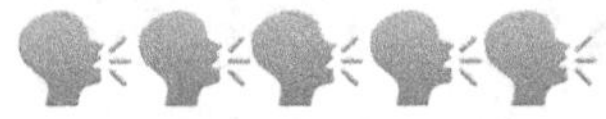

Valencia soon realized that if her grandfather had struggled with language as his disease progressed, other families must be facing the same barrier. Her grandfather didn't just speak English; he spoke French and Haitian Creole. This realization encouraged her to expand the project far beyond a simple English e-book. She knew that "Alzheimer's doesn't have a language barrier," and if she wanted her tool to be truly impactful, it needed to be accessible to diverse cultural communities.

She reached out to her friends and fellow students who were bilingual and asked them to volunteer their time to translate *Giselle Learns about Alzheimer's*. This led to a massive expansion of her outreach. Valencia hosted a dual-session day in Newark, New Jersey, where she spoke to the African American community in the morning and spent the afternoon with the Haitian community. During the afternoon session, a translator helped her communicate with the audience while they watched a YouTube video of the book being read in Haitian Creole. Seeing a room full of people finally understand the disease because the bridge had been built in their own language was a moment of "direct impact" that Valencia would never forget.

The project eventually reached the West Coast, where Valencia connected with girls in Arizona to hold additional virtual sessions. The measurable impact of her work was visible in the messages she received from people in their mid-40s who told her that the book had helped them, even if they didn't have young children. Valencia's project proved that a single story, when told with authenticity and translated with care, could dismantle mental health disparities and cultural stigmas. She had successfully turned a "small platform" into a national resource that allowed families of all backgrounds to see bits and pieces of themselves within the pages of Giselle's journey.

Beyond High School

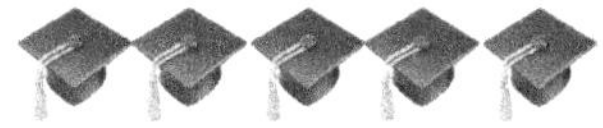

Completing her project was a "surreal moment" for Valencia, especially when she finally received the first 100 physical copies of her book. Opening that box in the house where all her memories of her grandfather lived was the happiest she had ever been. It served as "physical evidence" that she could accomplish anything she put her mind to. The project had transformed her from a shy freshman into a confident leader who knew how to ask for help and manage a complex team. She learned that being a leader doesn't mean doing everything yourself; it means knowing when to "fall back on those around you" and saying please and thank you to the village that helps you succeed.

The feeling of accomplishment she felt during her final ceremony, when she received her Gold Award pin and shook hands with her council leaders, "triumphed any feeling of stress" she had experienced during the project. Valencia hasn't left Giselle behind. She is currently working as quickly as she can to turn the book into a series. She believes that Giselle, as a diverse character, can help children learn about many other difficult topics, including the medical field, social history, and critical race theory. Valencia wants to take her small platform and "shine light in a new city" as she continues her studies and her advocacy work.

Valencia's advice to any girl who feels unmotivated during their own project is simple: the payoff is worth it. She encourages others to "take it, run with it, and fly as far as you can". Her own journey taught her that even the most devastating personal loss can be the fuel for a legacy that helps thousands of strangers. She started by trying to understand her grandfather's silence and ended by giving voice to a community that had been quiet for far too long. She proved that while a disease may steal a person's memory, it can never steal the impact of a girl with a mission and a book.

Chapter 7
Vision to Eye Health

Ifrah Attar (Ep 106)

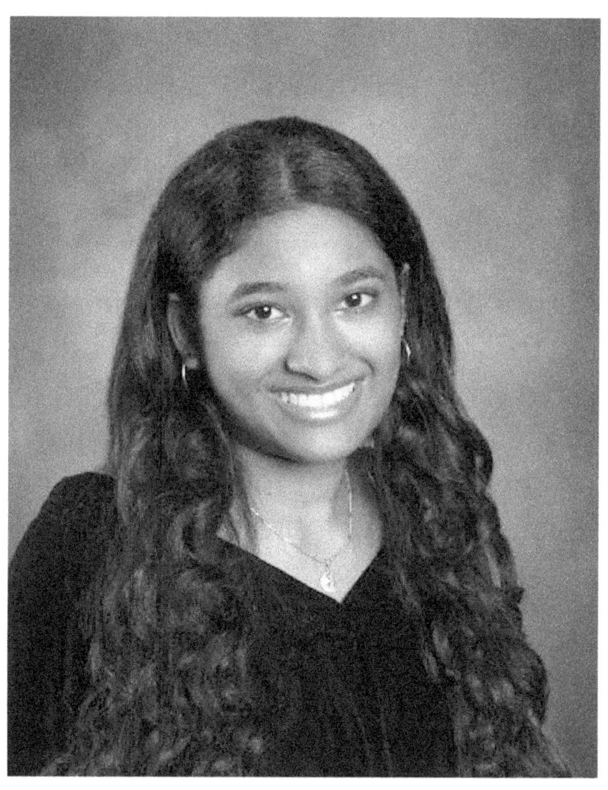

Blur That Changed Everything

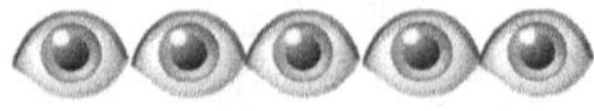

Ifrah Attar knew the world of blurriness all too well, having lived it every single day during her childhood. As a young girl, she frequently found herself sitting much too close to the television screen, her eyes straining to catch the details that her peers saw with ease. Despite the obvious signs that her vision was failing, Ifrah was a stubborn child who flatly refused to wear glasses or take the necessary steps to protect her eye health. This refusal was not just a phase but a lifestyle that she continued for years, unknowingly causing permanent changes to her physical sight. Eventually, the reality of her condition became impossible to ignore, and she was forced to start wearing glasses. Her personal experience highlighted a common community health issue-lack of awareness about eye care-that many children and families face, motivating her to take action.

While brainstorming for her Gold Award, Ifrah noticed a troubling trend in the news and medical reports. She discovered that since 2020, there had been a massive surge in child myopia cases across the entire nation. Experts were even going as far as to call this a "myopia crisis," as children were spending more time than ever before locked into digital screens. Ifrah realized that her own childhood mistakes were being repeated on a global scale by a new generation of kids who didn't know the risks. This realization hit her with incredible force because she knew exactly what it felt like to neglect your eyes. She saw a healthcare issue that simply was not getting the attention it deserved from parents or doctors.

Ifrah's motivation became a powerful combination of her own lived experience and her deep interest in advanced healthcare. She wanted to ensure that other children understood the importance of eye care before it was too late to reverse the damage. She knew that nearsightedness could affect a person for the rest of their life, impacting their education and their future career opportunities. Determined to bridge the gap between medical knowledge and family habits, she decided to launch her mission, which she titled "Child Myopia Awareness". She was ready to turn her personal regret into a public educational platform that could save the sight of hundreds of children.

Connecting Across the Miles

Turning a vision into reality required Ifrah to build a team of experts to help her navigate the complex world of ophthalmology. She knew that to be taken seriously by the community, she needed more than just her own story; she needed scientific backing. Her journey of connection began with her project mentor, Cheri Stewart, who served as a constant guide throughout the project. Cheri was the one

Ifrah turned to for suggestions, questions, and the critical networking connections needed to expand her reach. However, Ifrah wanted to reach even higher, so she decided to look for the top specialists in myopia.

While searching online, Ifrah came across the work of Dr. Terri Young, an ophthalmologist based in Wisconsin. Dr. Young was a world-renowned specialist with numerous publications on myopia, and Ifrah knew she was the perfect person to advise the project. The only problem was that Ifrah lived many states away, and reaching out to a professional of that caliber was incredibly nerve-wracking for a seventeen-year-old. Ifrah had to overcome her own anxiety and fear of rejection to format a professional email and hit the send button. To her delight, Dr. Young responded with enthusiasm, applauding Ifrah for her initiative and agreeing to serve as the project advisor.

This connection proved to be a turning point for the mission. Dr. Young provided Ifrah with a whole new perspective on her research, helping her move beyond preliminary facts into advanced medical insight. Ifrah learned that researching and finding emails and phone numbers was a skill that would serve her for the rest of her life. She didn't stop with Dr. Young; she also relied on her own family for support. Her parents offered creative suggestions on how to make the project look professional and engaging. Even her eight-year-old brother became a valuable team member, as Ifrah used him as a "test audience" to see if her presentations were easy for a child to understand. This diverse team gave her the confidence to move from the research phase into the heart of the community.

Blueprint for Better Sight

The core of Ifrah's project was a public community workshop designed to be both engaging and educational for children, parents, and educators. She knew that if she just lectured children, they would tune her out, so she filled her session with activities that made the science of the eye tangible. One of the most successful elements was a physical model of an eye that she used to demonstrate exactly how the eye stretches out when someone has myopia. Watching the children's eyes light up as they saw the mechanics of their own bodies was a rewarding experience for Ifrah. She also provided coloring pages and presentations filled with vivid pictures to keep the younger audience members focused and excited.

To ensure the project had a lasting impact, Ifrah created a tool that families could take home and use every day. Called the 'Eye Care Log,' it is a simple, easy-to-use booklet that encourages children to track their daily habits. The log helps children monitor three specific lifestyle changes that Ifrah found were most effective in preventing the myopia crisis: reducing screen time, eating leafy green vegetables, and spending more time outdoors. Through daily routines, the Eye Care Log makes eye health a shared responsibility, empowering children and parents to work together toward better vision.

To carry out the workshop and ensure the eye care habits became a permanent part of the children's lives, Ifrah utilized several key actions and tools:

- **Researched** the latest data on activities affecting eyesight to develop the three pillars of the Eye Care Log: reducing screen time, eating leafy green vegetables, and spending more time outdoors.
- **Developed** a creative curriculum that utilized hands-on models and interactive quizzes to show children how their daily habits physically changed the shape of their eyes.
- **Partnered** with the local library to secure a professional space for her community event, ensuring she had a trustworthy venue to host parents and children.
- **Rewarded** the students who completed their Eye Care Log for a full month with a gift card, providing a small incentive to help cement their new healthy habits.

Ifrah found that these incentives were a great way to keep the children motivated during the first month of their lifestyle changes. She made the log available for download so that even those who couldn't attend the workshop in person could still benefit from the project. The parents' feedback was just as positive as the kids'. Many parents admitted they had never realized their children were at risk and were grateful for the clear, actionable steps Ifrah provided. Ifrah was no longer just a teenager with a history of vision problems; she was a community educator providing a necessary service in a time of crisis.

Rolling with the Punches

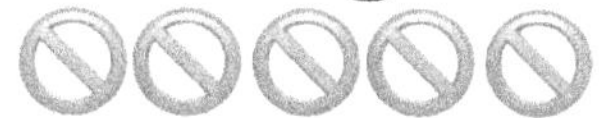

Even with a strong team and a great curriculum, Ifrah faced significant hurdles while trying to get her project off the ground. One of the biggest challenges was simply finding a location willing to host her workshop. Because she was only 17, many people in the community did not take her seriously and were hesitant to let her book a space for a public event. They saw her age as a barrier rather than a sign of her passion. Ifrah had to keep explaining her goal and her mission until she finally connected with the local library staff, who recognized the value of her work.

The second major hurdle was the project's timing, which coincided with the world still grappling with the effects of the pandemic. Ifrah found that many parents were still extremely hesitant to bring their children to a public indoor event. This fear of large gatherings meant that her marketing efforts had to be even more strategic. She spent hours creating eye-catching flyers and using social media to reach parents at home, explaining the safety measures she would take. Despite the uncertainty and the hurdles, Ifrah managed to get a good turnout of children, and the session went smoothly.

These challenges were not just obstacles to Ifrah; they were lessons in leadership and organization. She realized that she had to learn how to organize herself differently for her future, and that being a leader meant being the one to keep pushing when others said no. She had to be the voice that told herself she could do it, even when others put her down because of her age. Ifrah credited these difficult moments with helping her develop the resilience she would need for her future healthcare career. She learned that if a girl is passionate about her personal experience, that passion will shine through and convince others to join her cause.

Effect of a Single Voice

The impact of Ifrah's project began to grow in ways she never could have anticipated during the planning stages. During her workshop, a teacher from a local school attended the presentation and was blown away by the information Ifrah shared. She admitted that child myopia was an issue she had never truly considered before, and she asked Ifrah if she could take the project details to implement them into her own school and classroom. Having this type of response was a massive win for Ifrah, as it proved her project would continue to reach more kids, long after her work was done.

The most stunning moment of success came when Ifrah invited a state representative to attend one of her presentations. The representative was so impressed by Ifrah's research and her ability to connect with the audience that he gave her incredibly positive feedback. He suggested that Ifrah send him her project details so the Delaware Department of Education could use them across the entire state. Ifrah was overjoyed, feeling that all her hard work had truly paid off, as her message was now reaching thousands of people through the official education system. She had successfully moved the needle from a local workshop to a state-wide health initiative.

Ifrah's growth as a leader didn't stop with her project. She also founded a nutrition awareness club at her high school to address food insecurity and malnutrition among her peers. She realized that, just as with eye health, nutrition was a topic many high schoolers neglected because they were too busy or too tired to care. Through hygiene drives and making sandwiches for homeless shelters, Ifrah continued her legacy of service. She earned the Presidential Service Volunteer Award for her dedication to the community, having completed over 250 hours of volunteer work. Ifrah found that volunteering wasn't work for her; it was a stress reliever that she enjoyed doing with her friends and family.

Ifrah's future plans include advanced healthcare, where she hopes to develop medical devices and prosthetics. She encourages everyone starting a project to dive into their own past experiences to find their passion. She believes that if a project comes from a personal place, that drive will take you further than you ever thought possible. Her advice to anyone looking to make a difference is to never shy away from networking and reaching out to others, as those connections are the true engine of change. Ifrah Attar didn't just earn an award; she transformed her community's vision and ensured that the next generation would see a much brighter, clearer future.

Ifrah's project is like the careful grinding of a new lens for a world that has grown weary and out of focus: she realized that many were stumbling through a fog of digital screens and neglected habits, but by using the light of her own story, she polished away the blur of ignorance. Now, her work stands as a crystal-clear window, allowing children and parents to look toward the horizon with awareness and health, proving that when one girl chooses to focus her voice, she can improve the vision of an entire state.

Chapter 8
Running on Empty

Sarah Bland (Ep 135)

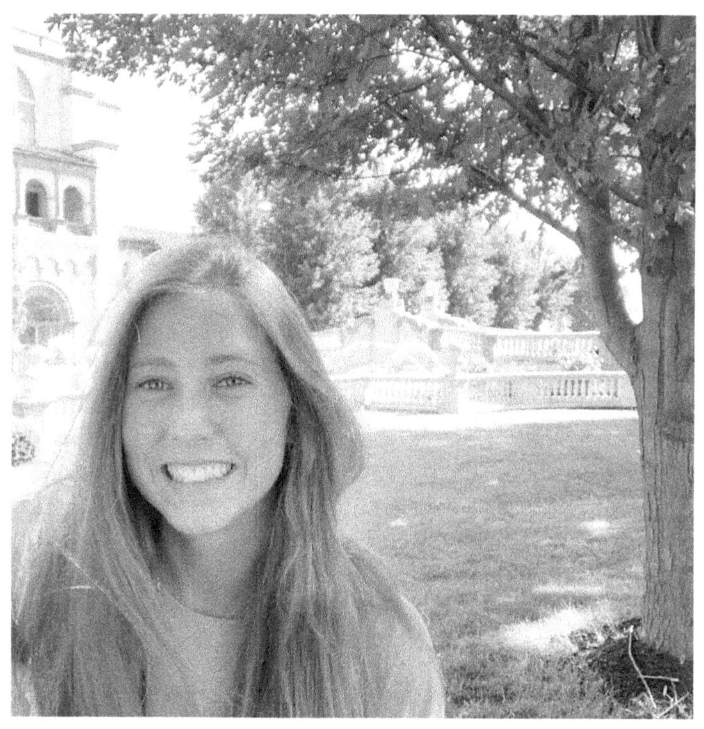

Invisible Anchor

Sarah Bland was always the girl you would see at the front of the pack. She lived for the sound of her spikes clicking against the track and the rhythmic thud of a soccer ball against her cleats. But during her junior year, something shifted that she couldn't quite explain. Her legs, which usually felt like coiled springs ready to explode, began to feel like heavy lead. Every workout became a grueling battle against a body that simply refused to cooperate. She was constantly tired, her focus in school was slipping, and she felt a strange lightheadedness every time she stood up too quickly. Her vision would sometimes even go black for a split second, a terrifying clue that something was wrong deep inside her system.

For a long time, Sarah tried to push through it, thinking she just needed more sleep or more "grit." However, her track coach noticed the change before she was even ready to admit it to herself. He pulled her aside after a particularly rough workout and said, "You're slowing down. You look fatigued in your workouts". He didn't just tell her to try harder; he gave her specific advice that would change the trajectory of her life. He recommended that she get her iron levels tested. When the results came back, the mystery was finally solved: Sarah was suffering from a significant iron deficiency.

The diagnosis was a relief, but the research that followed was a shock. Sarah discovered that she wasn't alone in this struggle. In fact, she learned that up to 35% of female athletes may experience this condition, yet it is often completely overlooked by doctors and coaches. Sarah realized that if a high-level athlete like her didn't know the signs, thousands of other girls were likely suffering in silence, thinking their lack of energy was just a personal failure. This realization became the spark for her mission. She decided to use her project to spread awareness about iron deficiency, ensuring that no other girl would have to run on empty without knowing why.

Global Hunt

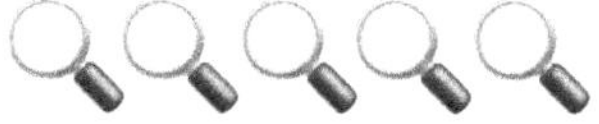

Sarah knew that if she wanted to change the minds of coaches and parents, she couldn't just speak from her own experience; she needed hard, scientific evidence. She began a deep dive into medical research that would eventually span over 200 hours. Her goal was to find a way to communicate complex medical facts so regular people—and especially busy athletes—could understand. She didn't just look at local resources; she searched for the world's leading experts on the subject.

During her online research, she stumbled across a groundbreaking article by a specialist named Dr.

Peter Peeling, who was based in Australia. Most high schoolers would be too intimidated to contact a world-renowned doctor on the other side of the planet, but Sarah was a girl with a mission. She drafted a professional email and sent it off, hoping for a response. To her delight, the connection worked. Dr. Peeling was impressed by her dedication, and after Sarah finished her research, he reviewed what she had put together and told her, "Wow, this is amazing." Having an international expert validate her work gave her the confidence she needed to push the project to its full potential.

Closer to home, Sarah built a support team that was just as powerful as her research. Her mother, who was highly skilled with technical tools, became her right-hand for the project's digital aspects. Her aunt, a doctor who was also an Ironman and ultramarathon runner, served as her official project advisor. Her aunt had experienced iron deficiency herself during her grueling races, so the project hit very close to home for her. Sarah was no longer just a student with a diagnosis; she was a leader preparing to educate her entire community. She was determined to bridge the gap between the medical world and the athletic field, turning "languishing" athletes into informed warriors.

Digital Blueprint

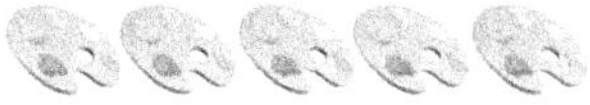

Carrying out a project of this scale required Sarah to master tools she had never even touched before. She realized that to reach the most people, she needed a central "hub" for all her information. This meant she had to learn how to build a website from scratch—a challenge she hadn't originally planned for but one she overcame through sheer persistence. She also knew that a long, dry report wouldn't grab a teenager's attention. She needed something visual, something that would pop.

Sarah turned to Canva to design a detailed infographic that distilled her hundreds of hours of research into a single, powerful page. She had to figure out how to pull out the most vital information, such as that standing up, seeing black, or losing concentration in school are major red flags. To make the information even more engaging, she used Doodly to create a 10-minute educational video. In the video, she used creative analogies, such as comparing a human body to a car that is slowly running down and losing its ability to drive.

The execution of the project involved many moving parts that Sarah had to juggle alongside her own busy schedule of track and school. To ensure her mission reached every corner of the community, she followed these specific steps:

Created a professional-grade website that served
as a permanent home for her findings,
allowing people to access the data even after
the project was officially over.
https://www.energetichealthyathlete.com/
Produced an interactive infographic on Canva that
highlighted the difference between heme iron
(from meat) and non-heme iron (from
vegetables) for different dietary needs.
Developed a Doodly animated film, which required
her to record and re-record her audio multiple
times to ensure her voice perfectly matched
the moving pictures on the screen.
Partnered with her school's track program to have
her website and infographics included in the
official parent and athlete manual given out
every season.

The process was far from easy. Sarah spent hours
syncing audio and fixing technical glitches on the
website. She learned that being a leader means
carving out the time to do the "tedious" work
because you are passionate about the end goal. By
the time she was finished, she hadn't just created a
report; she had built a digital legacy shared with
hundreds of athletes at summer camps and
through her school's athletic department.

Kitchen Science

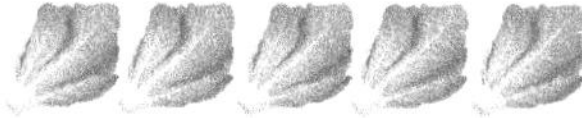

Sarah didn't want her project just to be a collection of websites and videos; she wanted to give people hands-on skills they could use in their daily lives. She knew that diet was the most effective way to manage iron levels, so she decided to lead a class for younger girls in her community. She wanted to show them that eating for strength didn't have to be boring or involve "disgusting" supplements. She wanted to show them that cooking could be a fun part of their athletic journey.

She developed a curriculum specifically for these younger girls, focusing on simple, delicious recipes rich in iron. Because the students were young, she kept the steps easy but focused on high-impact ingredients like spinach and turkey. They made what Sarah called "sushies," which weren't made with raw fish but were turkey-and-spinach wraps rolled into fun, bite-sized pieces. This approach allowed the girls to see spinach as an ingredient for strength rather than just a vegetable they were forced to eat.

One of the most important lessons Sarah shared in her kitchen classroom was the "citrus secret." She taught the girls that iron absorption is a complex process in the body, but there is a way to hack it. She explained that if you eat iron-rich foods—like spinach or turkey—alongside citrus fruits like oranges, your body can increase its iron absorption by up to six times. To put this into practice, they made smoothies that blended iron-rich leafy greens with bright, citrusy fruits. Watching the younger girls get excited about nutrition was one of Sarah's favorite parts of the entire project. She realized that by teaching them these habits now, she was preventing them from ever having to experience the "invisible lead" in their legs that she had fought against during her own junior year.

Crossing The Finish Line

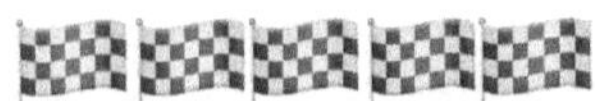

By the time Sarah received her final award, her project had reached far beyond her local track. She had received feedback from doctors across the community and had spoken to nearly 400 athletes at a major summer track camp. The project taught her something new about herself: she realized that once she put her mind to something, she could do it. When she was younger, the idea of completing a 200-hour leadership project seemed "crazy" and impossible, but she took it on and won.

The growth Sarah experienced as a leader translated directly into her future goals. As a high school senior, she began contacting college coaches to continue her track career. She didn't just send them her running times; she sent them her website and her research on iron deficiency. The coaches were incredibly impressed, and many of them reached back out to tell her that their own college programs required iron testing to keep their athletes safe. Sarah realized that her project had given her a "leg up" in the competitive world of college applications, showing that she was not just a runner, but a researcher and a leader in the health profession.

Sarah's advice to any other girl starting a big mission is to carve out the time and stay persistent. She learned that if you are truly passionate about your topic, the hours don't feel like a chore; they feel like an investment in your community. Sarah is looking forward to studying a health profession in college and continuing to run the sport she loves. Her journey proved that while iron might be a small mineral in the blood, a girl's voice is a powerful force that can move an entire community toward health.

Chapter 9
Knitted Friend

Noelle Buice (Ep 8)

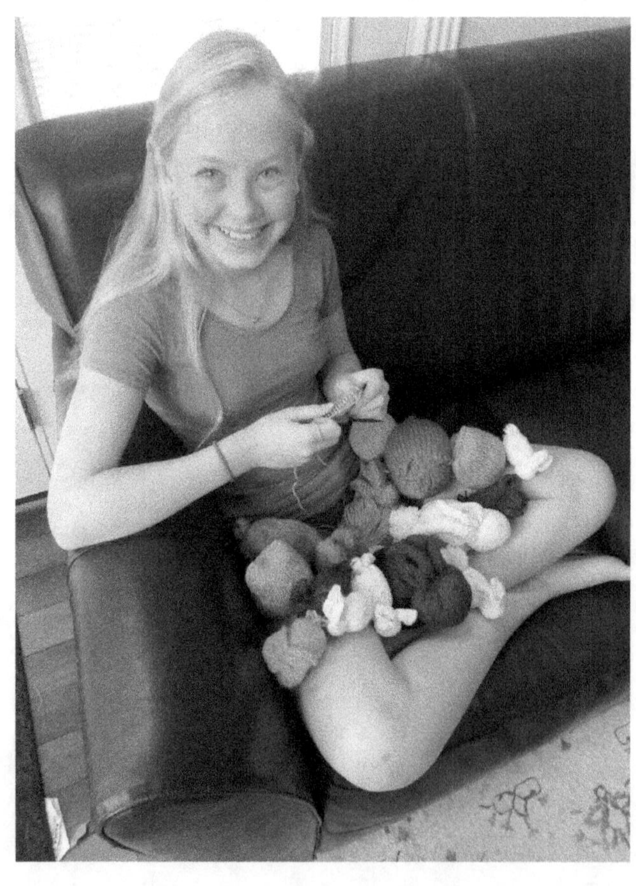

Quiet Power of a Soft Stitch

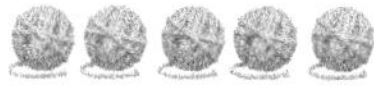

The year Noelle Buice entered the seventh grade; her world shifted in a way she never expected. While most of her classmates were worried about middle school lockers or upcoming math tests, Noelle was focused on a much heavier reality: her best friend had been diagnosed with cancer. The sterile, white walls of a hospital room are a difficult place for anyone, but for a young girl watching her friend battle a life-threatening illness, it was particularly devastating. Noelle knew she couldn't cure the disease, but she wanted to do something—anything—to bring a small spark of joy into that difficult space.

She turned to a skill she already loved: knitting. On the long drives to the hospital to visit her friend, Noelle's needles were constantly clicking away. She knitted several toys and stuffed animals, along with warm hats to help her friend feel cozy during her treatments. One day, Noelle looked at her friend's hospital bed and realized a surprising problem: the bed simply couldn't fit any more stuffed bunnies. The room was overflowing with soft, knitted comfort.

This "problem" of having too much kindness became the inspiration for something much bigger. Noelle looked around the ward and realized there were dozens of other children in the hospital fighting hard battles, often without a soft toy to hold on to. She began donating her stuffed animals to the other children in the facility. What started as a personal gesture for one friend quickly transformed into huge plastic bags full of stuffed animals being dropped off at the hospital doors.

As she transitioned into high school, Noelle realized this mission could reach far beyond her local area. She decided to launch a formal project called "Cancer Kicking Critters". She wanted to take what she had learned in middle school and expand it into a sustainable movement that could comfort children in dozens of hospitals. Her motivation was simple: if a "quirky fun thing" like knitting could make a difference for one friend, it could make a difference for thousands of children.

Nervous Silence

Scaling up a community effort into a major project required Noelle to develop a level of courage she didn't know she possessed. In the beginning, she was just a young student who was "nervous to talk to big groups of people" or get on the phone with strangers. She knew that to reach more children, she had to contact new hospitals and find volunteer groups to help her with the workload. The thought of calling a busy hospital administrator to ask if they would accept donations was intimidating.

Noelle's mother encouraged her to take the first step, reminding her that her cause was worth the momentary discomfort of a phone call. To her surprise, when Noelle finally began reaching out, the response was overwhelmingly positive. She discovered that people weren't judging her for being young; they were excited to help a girl who was so passionate about helping others. She learned that "everyone is very excited to help" and that the hardest part of any project is often just finding the bravery to ask.

Once she overcame her initial nerves, Noelle began visiting religious groups and community centers to find hands-on help. She attended church groups and even a synagogue, asking whether they had any knitting circles interested in donating simple knitted squares or completed toys. The community jumped at the chance to support her mission. One of her most dedicated partners became Miss Shirley Wallace, a volunteer who has since knitted several hundred octopi for the cause.

This phase of the project was about more than just toys; it was about building a network of support. Noelle learned that being a leader meant being a communicator and a recruiter. She realized that her passion for "Cancer Kicking Critters" was contagious. By sharing her story about her best friend and the stuffed bunnies, she recruited hundreds of knitters from all over the world, eager to contribute their time and talent to her growing organization.

Global Mission

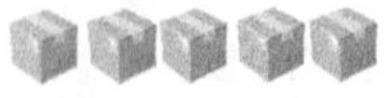

With hundreds of volunteers now sending in critters, Noelle had to manage the logistics of a worldwide operation. She didn't just want to hand out toys; she wanted the children in the hospitals to experience the joy of creation themselves. This led her to develop a unique system of kits. These kits allowed the children to take a simple knitted square and turn it into a bunny or another creature while sitting in their hospital beds.

Running "Cancer Kicking Critters" required Noelle to serve as a project manager, web designer, and fundraiser all at once. She launched a website, ckcritters.org, to track the organization's progress and share resources with volunteers. She even included a "critter count" at the top of the site to show exactly how many lives had been touched by the project. To keep the mission running smoothly, Noelle organized her efforts into several key areas:

Volunteer Outreach: She managed a network of hundreds of knitters and crocheters, including groups like "Kelly's Knits," who provided both finished critters and raw materials.

Resource Accessibility: She published 6 knitting patterns on her website, including a simple square, so volunteers of all skill levels could participate.

Kit Assembly: Noelle organized her team to package kits containing stuffing, eyes, and plastic bags, ensuring hospitals could easily distribute the kits to patients.

Financial Logistics: She collected monetary donations to cover the shipping costs of sending toys and kits to hospitals in faraway locations across the United States and Canada.

Noelle's team was a vital part of her success. Her mom served as a constant source of encouragement, while her aunt, who worked at Johns Hopkins, offered professional insight into hospital environments. Noelle had to learn how to balance all these moving parts with her own busy schedule. She was the captain of her high school rowing team, a leader in multiple choirs, and an active member of Young Life, her faith group.

She mastered the art of time management by fitting in work for her project and school whenever she could, ensuring that "Cancer Kicking Critters" never missed a beat. She learned that being a leader doesn't mean doing everything yourself; it means setting a vision and empowering others to help you reach it. By the time her formal project was complete, she had sent out 1,376 critters to children in need, proving that even a small hobby can have a massive impact when combined with organizational grit.

Curefest

As the project grew, Noelle began taking her mission to the national stage by attending Curefest in Washington, D.C. Curefest is a massive event where childhood cancer awareness programs, families, and organizations from all over the country gather to support one another. Noelle set up a booth and met with the parents and children who were directly impacted by the disease she was fighting through her critters. These interactions provided the most rewarding—and most difficult— moments of her entire journey.

The emotional toll of the project became real at these events. Noelle would return to Curefest year after year, sometimes seeing children who had improved and were now flourishing. "It was wonderful to see the ones that got better," she reflected. However, the experience was also "really emotionally tolling" because she would also meet parents whose children were no longer with them. Meeting the siblings of children she had met the previous year was particularly heartbreaking for Noelle.

These siblings would often tell Noelle stories about how they had sat in a hospital bed with their brother or sister, working on one of her kits to make a stuffed animal together. Hearing that her critters had provided a moment of connection and distraction during a family's darkest hours was a powerful reminder of why the work mattered. It transformed the project from a series of numbers on a website into a living legacy of empathy and love.

Despite the sadness, Noelle chose to focus on the "special light" the gifts brought into the children's lives. She learned to handle the heavy emotional weight of the project by focusing on the difference she was making in the present moment. She realized that she was helping families cope with the unthinkable, providing a soft, tangible reminder that they were not alone in their fight. This emotional resilience became a core part of her leadership growth, teaching her that true service often requires carrying the burdens of others with grace and strength.

Advocacy

Noelle's journey as a leader didn't stop with knitting; it opened doors to the highest levels of government. Through her project, she met with the head of the Environmental Protection Agency (EPA) to learn about science and environmental advocacy. She even had the opportunity to meet with Senators Warner and Kaine, speaking with them about legislation to increase funding for childhood cancer research. These experiences showed Noelle that a girl with a vision can influence the laws of the land.

The skills Noelle gained—time management, public speaking, and financial responsibility—have prepared her for whatever comes next. Whether she is leading her choir group, Rebel Trebles, or commanding her rowing crew as captain, she carries the confidence of someone who has already run a successful international nonprofit. She encourages other girls to jump into their own missions, telling them they can find any "quirky fun thing" they like and use it to change the world.

As Noelle looks toward her future, she remains dedicated to helping others. Her project taught her that you are never too young to start a movement and that a simple ball of yarn can be a lifeline for someone in need. She has proven that leadership isn't about the title you hold, but about the comfort you provide and the people you inspire to join you in the work. Noelle's story is a reminder that when we use our hands to serve, we strengthen the heart of our entire community.

Chapter 10
Dancing To Health

Parnika Saxena (Ep 32)

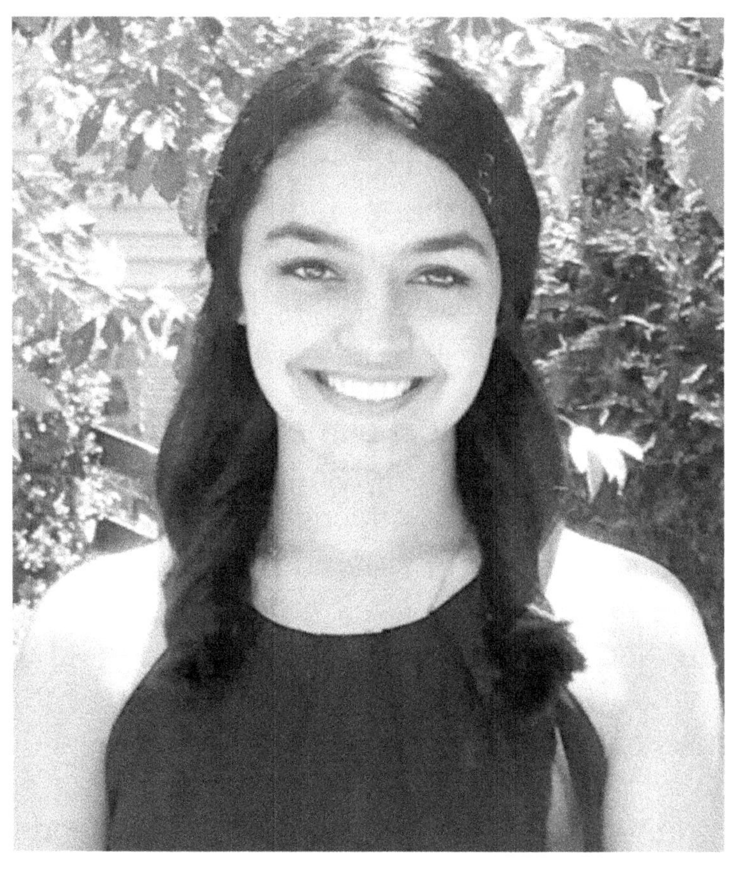

Rhythm of Heritage

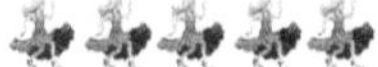

For Parnika Saxena, dance was not just a hobby; it was the language of her family. Growing up, she was surrounded by the rhythmic clicking of feet and the expressive storytelling of Kathak, a traditional Indian classical dance. Both her mother and her grandmother were dance teachers, and Parnika began her own training at the tender age of four. While other children were learning to ride bikes, Parnika was mastering intricate footwork and learning how to convey deep emotions through the movement of her hands and eyes. This passion became a core part of her identity, but as she grew older, she began to wonder how this ancient art form could do more than just entertain—she wanted to see if it could heal.

The spark for her project came from her own home. Parnika lived with all her grandparents, and she watched as they frequently visited the local senior center to socialize and stay active. She noticed how much they enjoyed being part of a community, but she also saw that many seniors struggled with isolation or physical limitations. She decided to use her skills to host dance workshops at the center, an initiative that served as the foundation for her early community work. The seniors absolutely loved it, and their enthusiastic response proved to Parnika that dance had a unique power to lift spirits and improve health.

Parnika knew she could take this vision even further. She didn't want to stop at one center or one age group. She wanted to explore the true scientific benefits of "dance therapy" on a massive scale. She realized that dance, as a form of exercise, triggers the release of endorphins—the brain's natural "happiness" chemicals. For her Gold Award project, she set out to bring this joy to people who were often overlooked: those in rehabilitation centers and students in her own high school. Her goal was to prove that you didn't need to be a professional athlete to be healthy and happy; you just needed to find your own rhythm.

Circle of Inclusion

As Parnika began planning the next phase of her project, she knew she had to adapt her beloved Kathak dance to fit the needs of everyone she met. It was one thing to teach a group of energetic children. Still, it was another challenge entirely to lead a workshop for people in rehabilitation centers, many of whom were in wheelchairs. Parnika refused to let physical constraints be a barrier to participation. She believed that everyone deserved to feel the "endorphin rush" that comes from movement, so she began stripping complex routines down to their simplest, most joyful parts.

She spent hours researching how to make her workshops inclusive. "I just wanted to focus on happiness," she explained, noting that her main goal was using dance to make everyone feel healthy and connected. For her senior and rehab participants, she shifted the focus from the feet to the upper body. She incorporated moves like "disco shakes" and simple hand gestures that everyone could do, regardless of their mobility. She even began selecting songs that her participants loved, blending traditional Indian music with their favorite tunes to get them "pumped and excited".

The project wasn't just about the physical workshops; it was about building a sustainable community within her own school. Parnika decided to start a dance club at her high school to ensure that her peers also had a creative outlet for their stress. She saw that high school could be an overwhelming environment, and she wanted to provide a "safe space" where students could laugh and move without judgment. By training others to lead these sessions, she ensured that the spirit of dance therapy would continue to grow long after she had moved on to the next stage of her life.

Leading the Movement

Executing a project that spanned multiple centers and schools required a high level of organizational skill. Parnika wasn't just a dancer anymore; she was a project manager, a recruiter, and a trainer. She had to coordinate schedules with multiple facilities, manage her own academic workload, and lead her team of volunteers through various sessions. The work was demanding, but seeing the immediate change in her participants made every minute of planning worth the effort.

The actual implementation of her project was a multi-step journey that combined her love for science with her artistic passion. To make sure the initiative was successful and reached the right people, she followed a very specific plan of action:

Adapted Choreography: She created specialized dance routines that focused on different body parts, such as arm-only dances for those with lower-body constraints.

High School Integration: She founded a formal dance club at her school, recruiting members and training them in the principles of dance therapy to ensure the program's sustainability.

Community Outreach: Parnika contacted local senior and rehabilitation centers to pitch her workshops, overcoming initial hesitation from staff and residents.

Resource Digitization: She began recording her adapted routines to create a library of videos that people could follow from the safety of their own homes.

One of the most rewarding parts of the project was watching the "visible difference" in the people she served. At the beginning of many sessions, the atmosphere was quiet and reserved. But as the music started and Parnika led them through the moves, the room would transform. "When you work with anyone, and you see them, the smile that comes onto their face is just an incredible feeling," she reflected. She wasn't just teaching a class; she was helping people interact with their friends and their environment in a new, more positive way. She proved that leadership is about empowering others to try something they've never done before.

Ripples

Every great leader face obstacles, and for Parnika, the biggest challenge was often the initial reaction of the people she was trying to help. When she first arrived at the senior and rehabilitation centers, she was met with doubtful stares. "What is this crazy young girl making us do these funny dance moves?" they would ask, wondering what good could come from a teenager's dance class. It took a great deal of patience and confidence for Parnika to stay the course. She had to use her communication skills to explain the benefits of her program and convince them that getting out of their "comfort zone" would be worth it in the end.

After a few sessions, the skepticism melted away. The seniors began looking forward to her visits, and their improved moods were a testament to the project's success. But Parnika's vision didn't stop at the borders of her town. She was fortunate enough to travel outside the United States and took her project with her. She expanded her workshops to a dance school in Dehradun, India, and even conducted a session in Kenya, Africa. These experiences gave her a unique global perspective on how happiness and movement are universal languages that tie people together regardless of their background.

In Kenya, Parnika had a truly unforgettable "full circle" moment. She met members of a Maasai tribe, and in a beautiful exchange of cultures, they taught her their traditional dances while she taught them her Kathak moves. However, the trip also taught her about the importance of sustainability. Because the village in Kenya lacked access to technology, she realized that her digital videos wouldn't work there. This led her to rethink how she could continue to support communities without high-tech resources. These global interactions taught her that while an idea might need to change to fit a new environment, the core goal of "enabling change" remains the same.

Becoming a Scientist

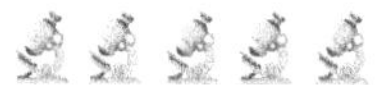

As Parnika's project reached its final stages, the world was suddenly hit by the pandemic. Parnika's leadership enabled development, allowing her to pivot to a new and urgent challenge. She was a member of her school's nanotechnology club, and she decided to apply her scientific research skills to the crisis. She began investigating a "super material" called graphene—an incredibly strong and lightweight form of carbon.

Parnika's new goal was to see if graphene could be used as a coating for face masks to prevent the spread of the virus. She researched a process called "nitrogen doping," which creates tiny pores in the graphene that allow oxygen to pass through but block virus particles. This was a "theoretical idea" that required intense research and outreach to professors and experts. Even though she was moving from the dance floor to the laboratory, the skills she learned during her project—patience, perseverance, and believing in herself—were exactly what she needed to tackle this complex problem.

Parnika is continuing her work on multiple fronts. She is developing a mobile app that uses a person's photo to identify their physical constraints and suggest adapted dance routines tailored to them. Reflecting on her journey, she realized that "any involvement with the community is incredibly fulfilling". She has transformed from a young girl learning dance steps into a visionary leader who uses both art and science to build a more inclusive and healthier world.

Chapter 11
Heart To Art

Angelica Arias (Ep 58)

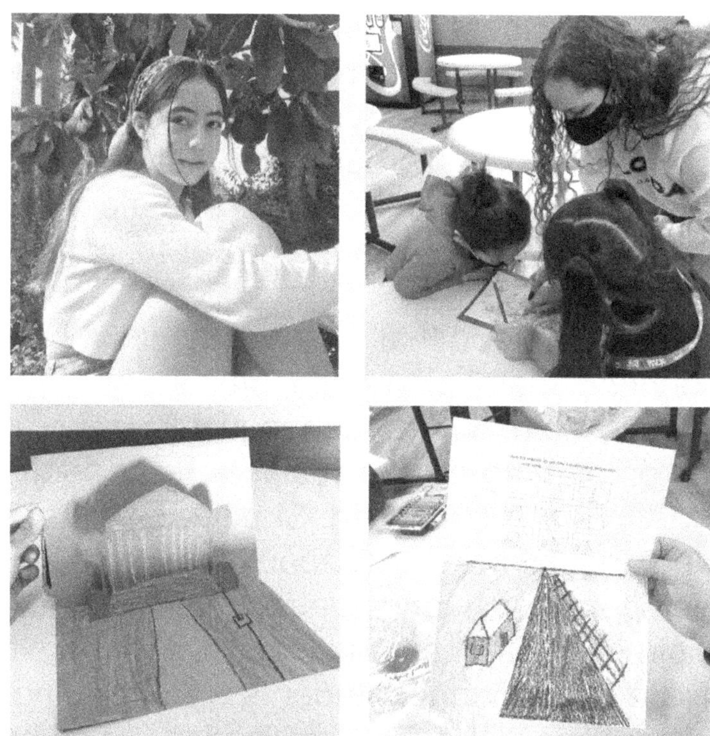

Vanishing Colors

Angelica Arias grew up in Broward County, Florida, where the sun usually shines bright, but she noticed a grey cloud looming over her local schools. The colors were literally fading from the classrooms. Because of a difficult budget situation, many public schools were cutting art programs and letting go of specialized art teachers. To some officials, art was just an extra, but to Angelica, it was a vital heartbeat of education. She knew that when you take away art, you don't just lose the chance to paint or sculpt; you lose a window into the rest of the world. Through her years as a Girl Scout, she had learned that if you see a problem in your community, you have the power to fix it.

Angelica understood that art education is a bridge that connects many different subjects. "Art education is so much more than just learning how to paint or learning how to sculpt or learn about color theory," she explained. She realized that by studying art, children learn about different cultures, complex geography, and even the social conditions of people in other times and places. It was a big deal to her that younger students were missing out on these connections. This realization fueled her passion to start a project she called "Heart to Art," an interactive enrichment program designed specifically for elementary schoolers.

She didn't want just to give the kids a one-time craft; she wanted to provide them with a mentor. She envisioned a program in which older students from her school, American Heritage, would serve as teachers. These club members would take a deep dive into specific art-historical periods and bring those stories to life for kids who might not even know what exists beyond Florida's borders. Her motivation was clear: she wanted to get the magic of learning back to her community and ensure that every child had a chance to see the world through a creative lens. She was ready to turn her passion into a movement that would paint a brighter future for her neighbors.

The Presentation Of A Lifetime

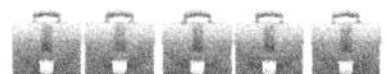

Before Angelica could help a single child, she had to navigate the professional world, which can be very intimidating for a high school student. Her first big hurdle was forming a partnership with a major community organization. She knew the Boys and Girls Club would be the perfect place to host her classes, but she couldn't just walk in the front door and start teaching. She had to act like a professional business leader. Early in high school, she requested a high-level meeting with the head of her own school.

The meeting was a major test of her confidence. "It was very scary because it was just me and I had to give this presentation to the head of my school," she recalled. She had to explain her vision, demonstrate that her project was sustainable, and establish a personal connection with the Boys and Girls Club's directors. Thankfully, the head of her school was impressed by her drive and her detailed plan. He put her in contact with Rich Olette, one of the directors of the Florence A. De George unit of the Boys and Girls Club.

But the work didn't stop there. Angelica had to secure a second meeting, this time with both the head of her school and Mr. Olette. She knew she couldn't just tell them the classes would be good; she had to show them. She spent weeks preparing a demonstration class, including a sample art project. This was her chance to practice her public speaking and prove that she could manage a group of students effectively. Her preparation paid off. Both leaders loved her demonstration, and they gave her the green light to bring her project to the club twice a month. This experience taught Angelica that even if something is scary, like standing in a room with powerful adults, having a well-researched plan gives you the strength to find your voice.

Designing The Masterpiece

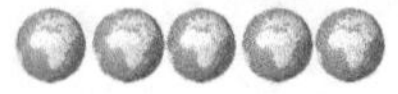

Once the partnership was official, Angelica had to transition from presenter to project manager. She founded the "Heart to Art" club at her school, and, to her delight, many other students eagerly joined. There were no special requirements to join; Angelica welcomed anyone with a passion for helping others, even if they weren't the best artists themselves. She organized bi-monthly Monday meetings to keep her team updated and ensure everyone was ready for their next teaching session.

The project was carried out with a very specific structure for every lesson to ensure the kids received a well-rounded education. Each club member took responsibility for one specific art period, researching its history and designing a curriculum. Angelica wanted the children to see the "bigger picture" of why art is made, so she made sure the lessons were much more than just a drawing tutorial. To make the learning process truly interactive and effective, she and her team followed these steps:

Global Introduction: They began each class by showing the kids the flags and the map of the country where the art period originated, discussing the languages spoken there.

Cultural Context: They explained the social conditions and events in the world at that time that inspired the artists.

Skill Application: After the history lesson, they led the students in a hands-on art project that allowed the kids to apply the characteristics and special details they had just learned.

Mentor Relationships: They focused on building a one-on-one connection with the children, acting as older siblings and guides throughout the process.

The reaction from the elementary students was immediate. They were incredibly curious about the world beyond Florida and loved seeing maps and hearing about other cultures. Angelica watched as the kids applied what they learned to their own projects. By teaching the "why" behind the "how," she was helping them develop a lifelong appreciation for history and global geography. Her project was no longer just an idea on a spreadsheet; it was a room full of children with paint on their hands and smiles on their faces, discovering that the world was much larger and more colorful than they had ever imagined.

Delivery Change

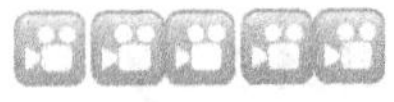

Just as Angelica's project was gaining momentum, she faced a challenge that changed the world: the pandemic. Suddenly, the "hands-on" and "up-close" nature of her program was a safety risk. She had to completely re-evaluate her dream of being in the classroom multiple times a month with dozens of children. For a moment, it was scary, and she wondered if she would have to scrap her entire project and start over.

With her family's support, she decided to reformulate the project rather than give up. She kept the core mission—teaching art and history—but pivoted to a hybrid model that included a heavy virtual component. Since no one could visit the Boys and Girls Club in person for a while, Angelica and her team started filming their lessons and posting them to Instagram and YouTube. This allowed her to reach even more children, as the links were sent via newsletters to kids in foster care through an organization called ChildNet.

When in-person classes finally returned, things looked very different. There were masks, social distancing, and a limit of only 10 students per session. The distance was difficult for Angelica because she knew how much the younger kids looked up to her and wanted to show her their work up close. "It's a little saddening," she said, but she quickly realized that "the magic is still there". The kids were so enthusiastic and excited to participate that even the masks couldn't hide their joy. She learned that a leader must be an innovator, finding ways to deliver a message even when global obstacles block the path. By embracing technology and staying flexible, she turned a pandemic hurdle into an opportunity to expand her reach to kids she might never have met in person.

A Legacy Beyond The Canvas

As Angelica reached the final stages of her project, she found that the most rewarding moments didn't happen during the lessons, but during the quiet times afterward. Her favorite memory was hearing the kids talk to each other while cleaning up the art room. One little girl told her friend, "Isn't this class so great? I love learning about history and doing a project after. It's so fun. I always look forward to it". Hearing those words made Angelica's heart feel "big and warm and fuzzy". She had succeeded in her mission to bring joy and knowledge to a generation left behind by budget cuts.

The project also transformed Angelica. She went from being an intimidated high schooler to a confident leader who could manage professional relationships and public speaking. She learned to organize her time between a grueling schedule that included the National Honor Society, horseback riding, and a difficult pre-law track at her school. "The project itself helped me break out of my shell," she realized, noting that the skills she earned are extraordinarily important for her life outside of school. She proved to herself that you don't have to spend five hours a day on a project to make a difference; just be consistent and tackle "those little achievements one at a time".

Looking toward her future, Angelica has a clear and unique path. She plans to attend college and then go to law school, but she wants to keep her creative side alive. She discovered a niche called fashion law, which perfectly blends her passion for the legal system with her love of design and fashion. She knows that the information she learned while building "Heart to Art" will never be lost. She encourages every girl on the edge of starting their own project to "just do it," because the relationships and the confidence you gain are more valuable than any award.

Angelica learned that leading a project is very much like painting a masterpiece. You start with a blank canvas of an idea, and sometimes the colors you planned to use aren't available, or the room's lighting changes unexpectedly. But if you have the patience to keep blending and the courage to try a new stroke, you can create something that is even more beautiful than you first imagined. Angelica didn't just teach a few art classes; she created a permanent gallery of hope in her students' hearts, proving that when a girl picks up a brush, she can change the world.

Chapter 12
Motherhood Matters

Megan Wang (Ep 45)

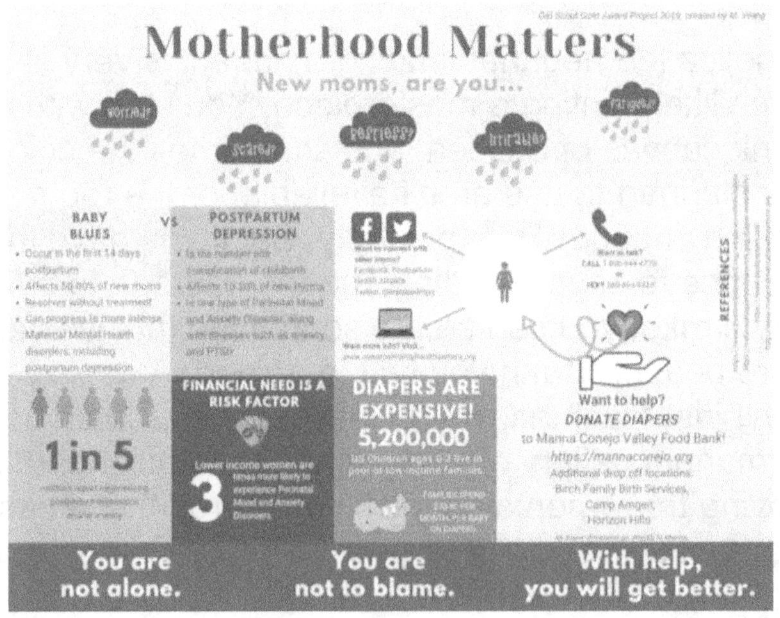

Spark In The Aisles

Megan Wang was a girl who understood the power of showing up for her community. For over twelve years, she had been a dedicated member of Girl Scouts, building a foundation of service that started with simple, heartfelt acts. One of her favorite memories involved the crisp November morning air during the yearly Veterans Day parades. She and her troop would march with pride, handing out pamphlets to the local heroes and even leading the crowd in the Pledge of Allegiance. These early experiences taught her that every small action contributes to a much larger picture of community well-being. However, it wasn't until she began her project in high school that she realized how many struggles in her own backyard were hidden in plain sight. Megan was searching for a way to make an "everlasting impact," and she found her calling while volunteering at a local food bank.

While guiding families through the food bank to pick out their monthly groceries, Megan noticed a recurring and heartbreaking pattern. Young mothers would frequently ask volunteers for diapers, only to be told the supply was low or exhausted. Diapers, something many people take for granted, were a luxury that many families simply couldn't afford. One conversation with a mother particularly moved her; the mom explained the crushing weight of financial stress she felt every day. She described how her childcare center was extremely costly and required families to provide a full day's worth of diapers for their child, even to attend. This requirement was a financial burden she couldn't always meet, leaving her trapped between the need to work and the inability to afford the basic supplies for her baby.

Megan realized that this wasn't just a physical problem of needing supplies; it was a spiritual crisis. "Talking with that mom made me wonder how financial difficulty can affect maternal mental health," she reflected. She saw the anxiety etched into the mothers' faces and knew she needed to do more than just hand out food. This moment was the "spark" for her project, which she would eventually name "Motherhood Matters". She decided to use her project to bridge the gap between financial stress and maternal well-being, ensuring that no mother in her community felt she had to carry the weight of the world alone.

Weight Of A Diaper

With a clear goal in mind, Megan began the extensive research and planning phase of her project. She knew that simply handing out diapers wouldn't be enough to create the sustainable change her project required. She needed to educate her community and provide long-term resources that would continue after her diaper drive ended. Megan spent weeks diving into the data, and what she found was staggering. She discovered that one in three families in the United States experiences "diaper need". Even more shocking was the fact that diapers can cost a family up to $960 per year. For a family already struggling to put food on the table, an extra thousand dollars is an impossible mountain to climb.

Megan realized that this financial strain was a direct trigger for mental health issues. She learned that one in five women reports experiencing postpartum anxiety and depression, yet it remains a "touchy topic" that many people are afraid to discuss. Megan noted that financial stress and the difficulty in providing necessities for a family can heavily impact a mother's mental state. She decided to split her project into two critical parts: a massive diaper drive and a wide-reaching educational campaign. Her project aimed to let mothers know they're not alone and that it's okay to ask for help, whether they're seeking diapers from the food bank or mental health resources.

To prepare for the education aspect, Megan researched maternal mental health and looked for ways to make help accessible. She didn't want the information to be buried in long articles that busy moms wouldn't have time to read. Instead, she focused on using technology to create a digital bridge to support. She looked to major organizations like Huggies, which offers excellent mental health resources on its website, and figured out how to direct families to those tools instantly. Megan was no longer just a high school student; she was becoming an advocate for 1,400 people who visit her local food bank every month. She was determined to ensure that every mother who walked through those doors felt seen and supported.

Ownership Speed Bump

Just as Megan was getting her project into high gear, she hit a major challenge that threatened her partnerships. She had arranged to work with three critical centers in her community: one birthing center and two childcare centers. These were the places where she would educate families through infographics and set up donation bins for outgrown diapers. She had spent months building a strong, responsive relationship with the original owner of the birthing center. This owner was incredibly supportive and knowledgeable about maternal mental health, making her a perfect partner for the mission. However, right in the middle of her project, the center underwent a sudden change in ownership.

Megan was not notified of this change, and she suddenly found herself trying to communicate with a new management team that was far less responsive. "That was a little speed bump in my project," she admitted. The new owners had multiple people managing their email accounts, leading to communication gaps and unanswered messages. Megan felt the pressure of her timeline slipping away as she waited for news on her donation bins. This moment could have discouraged any young leader, but Megan realized that "building a relationship" is the most important step in any collaboration. She learned that you can't just state facts; you need to build trust and persistence.

She refused to let the silence stop her. Megan continued to reach out politely but firmly, eventually clearing up the confusion with the new owners. This experience taught her that professional setbacks are often just tests of dedication. Beyond the logistical hurdle, she also had to navigate the sensitivity of her topic. Because mental health can be a "touchy topic," many people were initially hesitant to share their experiences. Megan matured as a communicator, learning that the best way to get people to talk about their mental health is to first build a genuine relationship with them. By overcoming the "speed bump" of the ownership change and the community's silence, she proved she had the resilience to lead a movement of care.

Assembly Line

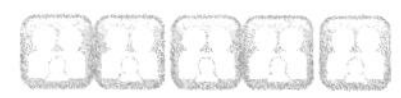

The project involved transforming Megan's home and partner centers into a professional-grade logistics operation. She gathered hundreds of diapers from the birthing center and childcare centers, but realized the food bank needed them sorted and packaged so they would be useful to families. Megan knew that the "team aspect" was a vital part of being a leader, so she reached out to younger girls in the program for support. Together, they turned a mountain of loose diapers into organized kits that were easy to distribute. Megan took great pride in the "education priority" of the work, ensuring that every package was more than just a donation.

Megan managed the execution of her project by breaking it down into several intentional steps:

Strategic Sizing: She sorted all the donated diapers into specific piles by size, from size one to size six, so that food bank workers could quickly find what a family needed.

Protective Packaging: She and her team of younger volunteers wrapped the diapers into uniform packs of exactly twenty using clean butcher paper.

Hand-Stamped Branding: The younger girls used handstamps to decorate the packages, giving the kits a personal, artistic touch that made them feel like gifts rather than just handouts.

Digital Integration: Megan affixed a QR code to the top of every single pack, which linked directly to an educational video she created about maternal mental health.

Watching the younger girls get excited about hand-stamping the packages was one of Megan's favorite parts of the journey. By involving them, she was passing on the spirit of service and teaching them that even simple supplies could be used to share important messages. The QR codes were the final, crucial piece of the puzzle. As mothers picked up diapers at the food bank, they were given instant, private access to a video explaining mental health resources and encouraging them to seek help if they were struggling. Megan had successfully combined a physical need with a digital solution, ensuring that her project provided "everlasting" support for the 1,400 people the food bank served each month.

Lasting Ripple Of Support

As Megan looked back on her finished project, the impact was visible in the relief of the mothers she served and the data from her local food bank. By providing thousands of diapers and a digital library of resources, she had given her community a permanent tool for wellness. The project had fundamentally changed Megan, as well. She realized that the skills she had built—researching maternal health, navigating changes in business ownership, and leading a team of volunteers—were tools she would carry into her future career. She learned that being a leader means focusing on the tiny details that others might overlook, like how a handstamp can make a donation feel more respectful.

After her project, Megan has a clear perspective for other girls who want to start their own journey. Her top piece of advice is to "start your project earlier in high school" so you can truly invest your time without the heavy workload of your final year. This allowed her to "focus on the details" and pour her heart into the mission. Even her fun personality stayed true throughout the process.

Megan is a girl who looked at a traditional problem and decided to simplify it, removing the "clutter" and focusing on the core essentials that really matter—comfort, dignity, and mental peace. Megan's journey shows us that a community is like a delicate garden. If the roots are struggling for basic needs like water or soil, the flowers cannot bloom. By providing diapers, she watered the roots of her community, and by providing mental health resources, she gave them the sunlight they needed to grow. Her story reminds us that when one girl finds her voice and refuses to let a "touchy topic" stay in the dark, she can light the way for thousands of others to find their own path to peace.

Chapter 13
Building Lifelong Wellness

Harvesting Lessons Of Health

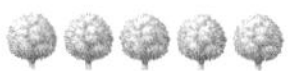

As you have traveled through the chapters of this book, you have witnessed a remarkable tapestry of leadership woven by young women who refused to accept the status quo in their communities' health. You read about the background of girls who faced devastating personal tragedies and turned that pain into a "Stress Less" sanctuary for their peers. You saw the challenge of "invisible anchors" like iron deficiency and rare diseases, and the action taken by leaders who became their own detectives to educate the world. You witnessed the impact of projects that provided 1,376 "critters" to hospitalized children and $52,000 for suicide prevention, proving that even "quirky fun things" like knitting or walking can change a community's trajectory.

The growth you observed in these pages is not just professional; it is deeply personal. These girls learned to manage "paperwork mountains," navigate the "clutter" of business ownership changes, and speak with confidence to Senators and school boards. They discovered that a project is not just a checklist to be completed, but a "living legacy" that continues to grow long after the final report is approved. They proved that "it is always perfectly okay to not be okay" and that seeking help is a sign of a strong leader, not a weak one. They moved from being girls with a mission to "lifelong changemakers" who carry the tools of resilience into their college years and careers.

Now, the baton is being passed to you. You have seen the "blueprint for change" used by those who cleared the air of vaping smoke and those who bridged the language barriers of Alzheimer's. You have learned the importance of "noticeable signals" and "academic grit". This next section is designed to transition you from a reader to a doer. It is your invitation to take the inspiration from these "Hearts of Gold" and apply it to a health issue that tugs at your own heart. Whether you are a student, a parent, or a community member, you possess the power to water the roots of your neighborhood and help it bloom.

Your Roadmap To Wellness

Building a health-related project is a journey that requires both a compassionate heart and a professional mindset. To help you navigate your own project, use the following steps as your guide, drawing on the wisdom of the leaders you have met:

- **Identify the Signals:** Look around your neighborhood or school. What is missing? Are people struggling with stress, a lack of supplies, or a "taboo" health topic? Focus on the "fundamental deficiencies" that need a solution.
- **Find Your "Why":** Why does this issue matter to you? Your passion will be the fuel you need when you face "paperwork mountains" or "speed bumps". As one leader noted, if you find your passion, the hours will go by in a flash.
- **Build Your Village:** You do not have to lead alone. Find an advisor—a teacher, a counselor, or a medical professional—who can provide guidance and moral support. Recruit a team of volunteers and learn to say "please" and "thank you" to the people who help you succeed.
- **Do the Deep Dive:** Become an expert on your topic. Spend the time researching so you can translate complex medical facts into language that regular people can understand. Reach out to experts, even if they are far away.
- **Embrace the Pivot:** Things will not always go according to plan. A true leader knows how to be flexible and innovative.
- **Create for Sustainability:** How will your work continue after you finish? Design digital

hubs, write books, or create "kits" and "manuals" that others can use long after your project is complete.

As you step out to lead, remember the "ripple effect". Your decision to address one small problem can lead to a national movement or a "thank you" from a little girl on a bus who found a daily healthy habit because of you. The payoff is worth every sacrifice. Take your unique gifts, follow your heart, and "run with it and fly as far as you can". Your story is the next chapter in the legacy of health and wellness.

ABOUT THE AUTHOR

Sheryl M. Robinson is a podcaster, mentor, and speaker dedicated to helping teens and young adults discover their unique gifts, talents, and abilities, creating a path toward their dreams.

Sheryl holds a Master of Arts in Servant Leadership from Viterbo University and a Bachelor's in Accounting from Southern Illinois University – Carbondale. She has been a proud member of Girl Scouts for more than 30 years. Her passion for supporting teens — especially those pursuing the Girl Scout Gold Award — led her to create *Hearts of Gold*, a YouTube series and podcast featuring Gold Award Girl Scouts from across the world.

In recognition of her work elevating and supporting the Girl Scout Highest Awards, Sheryl has been honored with the GSUSA Thanks II Award, the organization's highest recognition for service.

Recognizing the need for younger Girl Scouts to have resources and role models as they pursue the Bronze Award and Silver Award, Sheryl created this middle-grade book series to share inspiring stories of leadership, courage, and community change.

She deeply believes that the Girl Scout Highest Awards not only make the world a better place but also transform the Girl Scouts who earn them — building lifelong changemakers, confident problem-solvers, and compassionate leaders.

ACKNOWLEDGMENTS

Creating this book has been a journey shaped by many remarkable people, and I am deeply grateful for each of you.

To **my mom, Jean**, who first started me in Girl Scouts many years ago and planted the seeds of everything that would follow.

To **my daughter, Nikki**, a Bronze, Silver, and Gold Award Girl Scout whose dedication inspires me every day. Watching you flourish through each phase of your life is one of my greatest joys.

To **my husband, Mark,** thank you for always supporting me and the many plates you quietly set beside me while I typed away. I thank God for bringing you into my life every day.

To **Calley and Eloise,** thank you for reading the first draft and sharing thoughtful feedback. Your insights helped shape this book and made it stronger.

To **all the Gold Award Girl Scouts** who have shared their stories on the Hearts of Gold podcast — thank you for trusting me with your journeys. Your courage, creativity, and leadership inspire thousands.

To the **Girl Scout leaders, volunteers, and parents** who support these incredible young women: your encouragement makes meaningful change possible.

To **Cassie**, who encouraged me to restart my Girl Scout journey when my daughter joined Girl Scouts.

A heartfelt thank you to **Stacie and Shannan**, who have listened to me talk about this book for years and never stopped encouraging me to make it happen.

To **Walter**, my podcast editor for the first nine years, and **Tommy**, my new editor — and to their entire family, especially **Greg**, whose podcasting challenge a decade ago helped set all of this into motion.

And finally, to **Elsie, Rob, Cliff, Daniel, and Jessica** — thank you for your inspiration, for keeping the process fun, for sharing your knowledge, and for helping Hearts of Gold continue to grow.

This project exists because of each of you.
Thank you for helping bring these stories to life.

To all the future Bronze, Silver, and Gold Award Girl Scouts and others inspired by this book – Be the change you want to see in the world and remember <u>your</u> leadership matters.

MORE STORIES

Want to hear more inspiring stories from Gold Award Girl Scouts?

HeartsofGoldPodcast.com

You can watch or listen to new episodes every month.

Podcast:
https://bit.ly/3JT7x0w

YouTube:
https://bit.ly/3P5nns8

Instagram:
https://bit.ly/3JZ2JX8

www.ingramcontent.com/pod-product-compliance
Lightning Source LLC
Chambersburg PA
CBHW050953050726

47592CB00007B/2557